西藏与新疆地区慢性心肺疾病现状调查项目论文集

王增武　主编

中国协和医科大学出版社

图书在版编目（CIP）数据

西藏与新疆地区慢性心肺疾病现状调查项目论文集 / 王增武主编. —北京：中国协和医科大学出版社，2019.4

ISBN 978-7-5679-1232-8

Ⅰ.①西… Ⅱ.①王… Ⅲ.①心脏血管疾病-慢性病-调查研究-西藏-文集 ②心脏血管疾病-慢性病-调查研究-新疆-文集 ③肺疾病-慢性病-调查研究-西藏-文集 ④肺疾病-慢性病-调查研究-新疆-文集 Ⅳ.①R54-53 ②R563-53

中国版本图书馆 CIP 数据核字（2019）第 013121 号

西藏与新疆地区慢性心肺疾病现状调查项目论文集

主　　编：王增武

责任编辑：顾良军

出版发行：**中国协和医科大学出版社**

（北京东单三条九号　邮编 100730　电话 65260431）

网　　址：www.pumcp.com

经　　销：新华书店总店北京发行所

印　　刷：北京朝阳印刷厂有限责任公司

开　　本：787×1092　1/16

印　　张：13.25

字　　数：260 千字

版　　次：2019 年 4 月第 1 版

印　　次：2019 年 4 月第 1 次印刷

定　　价：96.00 元

ISBN 978-7-5679-1232-8

编委会成员名单

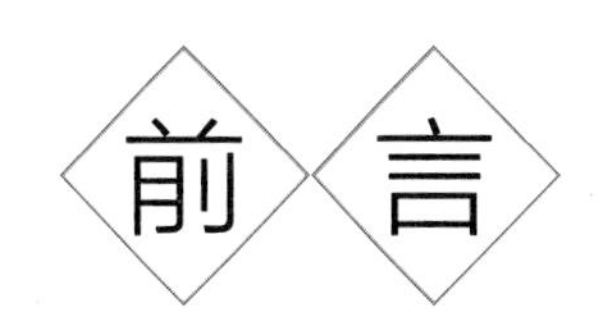

前言

“西藏与新疆地区慢性心肺疾病现状调查研究”由原国家卫生与计划生育委员会立项，是一项惠及多民族群众的公益项目。2014年制订方案；到2017年4月，在原国家卫计委、原解放军总后勤部和西藏、新疆卫计委的领导下，该项目由国家心血管病中心联合北京医院、中国疾病预防控制中心、中国人民解放军总医院、新疆维吾尔自治区人民医院等单位带动基层、社区行政和医疗机构协同完成。

参加项目的医务人员和科研工作者认真总结归纳，潜心分析研究，形成科研成果。本书所选录的18篇论文和10篇会议摘要，是这项活动的优秀科研成果。科研人员即论文作者，在不同地区、不同岗位，全部参加了一线调查研究，为本书科研成果的形成提供了宝贵的资料。纵观本书，有以下特点。

首先，科研人员具有高度的事业心和责任感。本项目调查涵盖新疆7个区县、西藏6个区县。西部地区特殊的地理环境和气候条件给调查带来了难以想象的困难。科研人员与医务工作者克服恶劣的自然条件，坚持完成了复杂而繁重的实地调查任务，并对相关病人进行后续帮扶与治疗。在艰苦细致的调查中，科研人员满怀高度的事业心和责任感，白天工作，晚上归纳研究。他们忍着高原反应和沙漠高温，夜以继日地调查，马不停蹄地研究，回到北京、拉萨、乌鲁木齐或在地方上，继续全身心地扑在科研上，分析数据，研究病例，旁征博引，撰写论文，形成今天的成果。

二是论文水平高，学术价值大。本书共分两部分，一部分为论文，另一部分为会议摘要，后者主要记录了该调查项目及论文在不同论坛上发表和交流的情况。17篇论文中，反映疾病防控的占14篇，反映基层医疗环境、专业配置的占4篇。反应疾病防控的论文涉及多种心肺疾病在西藏和新疆的流行状况调查，范围包括高血压、慢性阻塞性肺疾病、支气管哮喘、慢性肺源性心脏病、超重/肥胖、糖尿病、血脂异常、心房颤动、慢性心力衰竭、瓣膜性心脏病、高原性心脏病、外周动脉疾病、先天性心脏病等。在大量调查数据基础上，科研人员进行了全面系统的分析研究。入选本书的论文大部分已经发表，并在国内国际专业会议、论坛上进行了交流，其中至少有10篇论文在第四届世界高血压大会、第19届中国南方国际心血管病学术会议和中国心脏大会上进行了交流。这些论文建立在大量科学调查数据基础之上，具有较高的学术价值，引起与会专家和国家、地方有关部门的高度重视。

三是贴近实际，有重大的现实意义。这次专项调查地域广，人口覆盖面大。其中，新疆维吾尔自治区调查15岁以上居民共7 394人，西藏自治区调查15岁以上居民共5 801人。因此，调查积累了大量一手资料。论文以多民族群众的专项健康调查数据为研究对象，注重实地和实际。例如,《西藏不同海拔地区高血压患病情况调查》以海拔高度划分研究人群;《新疆和西藏地区居民体重指数及腰围与10年冠状动脉粥样硬化性心脏病发病风险的关系》以地域身体特征和发病区间进行比较研究。因此，这些论文具有很强的地域性、族群针对性和说服力，加大了科研含量，增强了群众防治肺心病的意识。本项目是一项公益性质的科研活动，全面准确掌握了新疆、西藏地区居民慢性心肺疾病及主要危险因素的流行现状。因此，这些论文既是科研成果，又是国家和地方进行科学决策的依据，有利于国家和地区制定科学、可行的疾病防治规划和策略，有效预防和控制慢性心肺疾病，减少其对西藏和新疆居民健康的危害。

人民健康是民族昌盛和国家富强的重要标志。十九大后的首次国家科技奖励大会上，中国疾病预防控制中心病毒病预防控制所侯云德院士获得国家最高科学技术奖，这充分体现了党和国家对人民健康事业的关心和重视。我们希望收集编纂的这些专项论文成果，能对促进我国西部地区乃至全国群众的健康起到积极作用。当然，这些论文仅是这个调查项目的部分成果；随着分析研究的深入，我们相信，将会有更多的成果呈现给大家。

说明：此项调查研究均原自公益性行业专项“西藏与新疆地区慢性心肺疾病现状调查研究”（编号201402002）专项基金，故正文中均不再列出资金来源。

编者

2019年1月

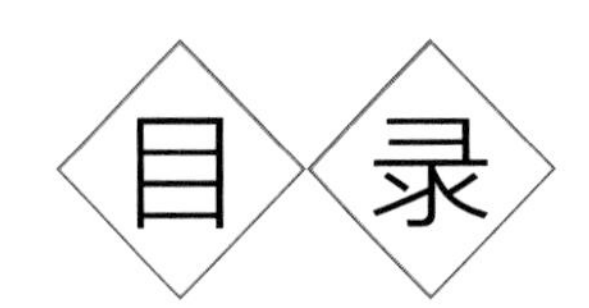

已发表论文

会议论文摘要

已发表论文

西藏新疆地区静息心率与血脂、血糖的关系研究△

王增武，陈　祚，王　馨，张林峰，郝　光，董　莹，聂静雨，王佳丽，郑聪毅，邵　澜，田　野

中国医学科学院阜外医院，国家心血管病中心社区防治部　北京 . 102308

通讯作者：王增武，E-mail：wangzengwu@foxmail.com

摘　要　目的　探索西藏和新疆地区心率和血脂、血糖的关系。**方法**　2015～2016 年期间，用分层多阶段随机抽样，选取西藏新疆地区 35 岁及以上调查对象 7 510 人，有效数据 5 477 人。利用该资料分析心率和血脂、血糖的关系。**结果**　发现随着心率的增加血脂异常和糖尿病的患病风险随之增加（多因素分析调整年龄、性别、民族、体重指数、吸烟、饮酒、教育程度、高血压和居住海拔后 $P < 0.05$，心率最高三分位数组到最低三分位数组的血脂异常患病率为 16.0%、19.4% 和 19.9%；糖尿病的患病率为 2.2%、3.0% 和 5.2%。使用一般线性回归分析调整年龄、性别、民族、体重指数、吸烟、饮酒、教育程度、高血压和居住海拔后发现 TC（$\beta=0.003$，$P<0.05$）、TG（$\beta=0.005$，$P<0.05$）和血糖水平（$\beta=0.009$，$P<0.05$）和心率成正相关。本研究并未发现心率和居住海拔之间对血脂、血糖的影响存在交互作用（$P>0.05$）。**结论**　本研究发现心率与血脂、血糖水平呈正相关，心率和居住海拔之间对血脂、血糖的影响无交互作用。

关键词　心率；血脂；血糖；相关关系；交互作用

The Associations of Resting Heart Rate with Plasma Lipid Profiles and Blood Glucose in Tibet and Xinjiang

Wang Zengwu, Chen Zuo, Wang Xin, Zhang Linfeng, Hao Guang, Dong Ying, Nie Jingyu, Wang Jiali, Zheng Congyi, Shao Lan, Tian Ye.

National Center for Cardiovascular Diseases & Fuwai Hospital, CAMS and FUMC, Beijing

△　本文发表于：心脑血管病防治，2017，17（2）：89-92.

102308, China

Abstract　Objective　To examine the association between heart rate, blood lipid profiles and blood glucose among Tibetan and Xinjiang population. **Methods**　Using stratified multi-stage random sampling, 7 510 residents aged 35 or older were detected with international standardized examination in Tibet and Xinjiang during 2015 ~ 2016. At length, there were 5 477 participants were eligible for the analysis. **Results**　After adjustments for age, gender, race, body mass index, smoking, alcohol consumption, education, hypertension, and the altitude of habitation, the multivariate analysis found that the higher heart rate was significantly associated with dyslipidemia and diabetes. The percentage of dyslipidemia in tertile 1, tertile 2 and tertile 3 of heart rate were 16.0%, 19.4%, and 19.9%, while the percentage of diabetes were 2.2%, 3.0%, and 5.2%, respectively. After adjustments for age, gender, race, body mass index, smoking, alcohol consumption, education, hypertension and the altitude of habitation, the general linear regression analysis revealed that total cholesterol (TC) (β = 0.003, $P < 0.05$) and triglyceride (TG) (β = 0.005, $P < 0.05$) was positively associated with blood glucose (β = 0.009, $P < 0.05$)and heart rate. There was no interaction between heart rate and altitude of habitation ($P > 0.05$) on the blood lipid profiles and blood glucose. **Conclusions**　The heart rate is positively associated with dyslipidemia and diabetes. However, there is no interaction between heart rate and altitude of habitation on the blood lipid profiles and blood glucose.

Key words　Heart rate; Lipid profiles; Blood glucose; Association; Interaction

血脂异常和糖尿病是最常见的慢性病，也是心脑血管病最主要的危险因素，严重消耗医疗和社会资源，给家庭和国家造成沉重负担[1, 2]。随着我国经济水平的发展，人们生活水平普遍提高，血脂异常和糖尿病及其导致的心血管疾病患病率有逐年上升的趋势[3]。心率可以反映自主神经系统活性和评估心脏交感神经与迷走神经张力及其平衡性，因此可能作为心脏代谢性疾病的预测因子[4, 5]。国内外关于心率对糖尿病、血脂异常的研究结论存在争议[6 ~ 9]。另外目前缺乏基于居住在不同海拔人群的相关研究[8]。因此，本研究使用西藏与新疆地区慢性心肺疾病现状调查研究数据探索心率和血脂、血糖的关系，同时探索心率与居住海拔对血脂、血糖水平的影响是否存在交互作用。本研究结果可以丰富对血脂异常和糖尿病影响因素的认识，为预防干预策略的制定提供一定依据。

1. 对象和方法

1.1　研究对象

本次调查采用分层多阶段随机抽样。首先分别在西藏和新疆自治区内按城乡分为 2 层，在每层内采用与容量大小成比例的概率（probability proportional to size，PPS）抽取所需数量的区 / 县。然后在每个被抽中的区 / 县中采用简单随机抽样（simple random sampling，SRS）方法抽取 2 个街道 / 乡镇。再在每个被抽中的街道 / 乡镇中采用 SRS 法抽取 3 个居委会 / 村委会。最后在被抽中的居委会 / 村委会中分性别、年龄采用 SRS 方法随机抽取调查个体。实际入选 35 岁调查对象 7 510 人，有效数据 5 477 人。本项研究通过中国医学科学院阜外心血管病医院伦理委员会批准，所有参加对象均签署知情同意书。

1.2　研究方法

调查人群采用统一的调查方案、调查手册及调查问卷。各人群的主要调查人员、质控人员以及资料录入人员在调查前均进行培训并通过考核。问卷内容包括一般人口学特征、家庭年收入及疾病史。血压和心率的测量采用电子血压计（Omron HBP-1300），连续测 3 次，每次至少间隔 30 秒，取 3 次读数的平均值为个体血压值。每位参加者静坐休息 5 分钟后测量血压，测量前半小时内避免吸烟、饮酒、饮用含有咖啡因的饮料以及剧烈运动。体重和身高进行两次测量。测量体重时要求空腹，只穿轻薄衣物、脱鞋，精确至 0.1kg 测量身高时脱鞋，精确至 1mm。体重指数（BMI）为体重（kg）除以身高平方（m^2）。

采取空腹 12 小时血标本用于测定血脂、血糖等生化指标。所有标本先保存于 －70℃冰箱，标本采集完成后由统一实验室进行检测。所有生化检查采用美国贝克曼库尔特有限公司（Beckman Coulter，Inc.）AU400 自动生化分析仪，试剂也为该公司制作。血糖、血脂应用酶法测定。

1.3　诊断标准

高血压诊断标准采用2004年《中国高血压防治指南》推荐的标准：收缩压 ≥ 140 mmHg 或舒张压 ≥ 90 mmHg，对既往确诊的高血压患者或在两周内服用过降压药者，不论检查时血压是否异常均诊断为高血压。糖尿病定义为既往确诊或实验室检查空腹血糖 ≥ 7.0 mmol/L。血脂异常定义为 TC ≥ 6.22 mmol/L、TG ≥ 2.26 mmol/L、HDL-C < 1.04 mmol/L、LDL-C ≥ 4.14 mmol/L 和 / 或两周内服用降脂药。吸烟者定义为一生中至少吸过 20 包烟且最近一个月仍在吸烟。饮酒定义为最近一个月每周至少饮酒一次。

1.4　统计学处理

采用 SPSS16.0 软件进行统计学分析。计量资料用（$\bar{X} \pm s$）表示，两组间比较用 t 检验；两组率的比较用 χ^2 检验。危险因素分析采用一般线性回归模型。$P < 0.05$ 为差异有统计学意义。

2. 结果

2.1 基本情况

本次调查纳入 7 510 名调查对象，5 477 有效数据用于此研究分析，其中男性 2 425 人（44.2%），女性 3 052 人（55.7%）。女性中 BMI 水平、心率、汉族人群及居住海拔高的比例高于男性。男性的吸烟 / 饮酒率、初中及以上教育程度及糖尿病的比例均明显高于女性（$P < 0.05$）。其他特征两组之间差异无统计学意义（$P > 0.05$），见表 1。

表 1 研究对象的一般特征

特　征	男性（n = 2 425）	女性（n = 3 052）	合计（n = 5 477）	*P*
年龄（岁）	53.6 ± 13.0	53 ± 12.2	53.3 ± 12.6	>0 05
民族（汉族）	1 018（42.0）	937（30.7）	1 955（35.7）	<0.01
体重指数（kg/m^2）	25.4 ± 3.8	25.6 ± 4.2	2 5.5 ± 4.0	>0.05
吸烟（%）	965（39.8）	106（3.5）	1 071（19.6）	<0.01
饮酒（%）	438（18.1）	99（3.2）	537（9.8）	<0.01
教育程度（初中及以上，%）	1 019（42）	924（30.3）	1 943（35.5）	<0.01
高血压（%）	827（34.1）	994（32.6）	1 821（33.2）	>0.05
心率（次 / 秒）	75.3 ± 11.6	76.5 ± 11	75.9 ± 11.3	<0.01
居住地海拔（m）				
<1 000	1 215（50.1）	1 309（42.9）	2 524（46.1）	<0.01
1 000 ~ 3 500	861（35.5）	1 039（34.0）	1 900（34.7）	
≥3 500	349（14.4）	704（23.1）	1 053（19.2）	

2.2 糖尿病及血脂异常患病情况

本研究发现随着心率的增加血脂异常和糖尿病的患病风险随之增加（多因素分析调整年龄、性别、民族、BMI、吸烟、饮酒、教育程度、高血压和居住地海拔高度，$P < 0.05$），心率最高三分位数组到最低三分位数组的血脂异常患病率为 16.0%、19.4% 和 19.9%；糖尿病的患病率为 2.2%、3.0% 和 5.2%（图 1、图 2）。

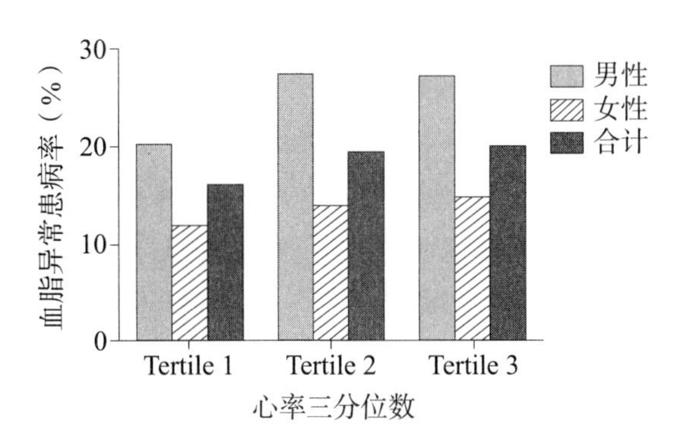

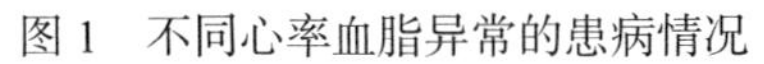
图1　不同心率血脂异常的患病情况

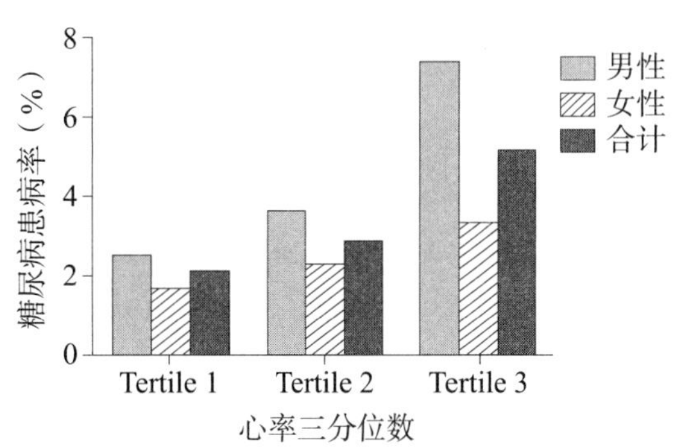

图2　不同心率糖尿病的患病情况

2.3　血脂、血糖水平的多因素分析

使用一般线性回归分析调整年龄、性别及民族后发现 TC（β = 0.004，$P < 0.05$）、TG（β = 0.01，$P < 0.05$）和血糖水平（β = 0.009，$P < 0.05$）与心率成正相关。进一步调整 BMI、吸烟、饮酒、教育程度、高血压和居住海拔后相关性仍具有统计学意义（TC：β = 0.003，$P < 0.05$；TG：β = 0.005，$P < 0.05$；血糖水平：β = 0.009，$P < 0.05$）（表2、表3）。本研究并未发现心率和居住海拔之间对于血脂、血糖的影响存在交互作用（$P > 0.05$）。

表2　研究对象血脂、血糖水平

特　征	男性（n = 2 425）	女性（n = 3 052）	合计（n = 5 477）	*P*
血糖（mmol/L）	5.3 ± 1.5	5.0 ± 1.1	5.1 ± 1.3	< 0.01
TC（mmol/L）	4.6 ± 0.9	4.7 ± 1.0	4.7 ± 0.9	> 0.05
TG（mmol/ L）	1.3 ± 1.0	1.0 ± 0.6	1.1 ± 0.8	< 0.01
HDL-C（mmol/L）	1.3 ± 0.3	1.5 ± 0.3	1.4 ± 0.3	< 0.01
LDL-C（mmol/L）	2.7 ± 0.8	2.7 ± 0.8	2.7 ± 0.8	> 0.05

TC，总胆固醇；TG，甘油三酯；HDL-C，高密度脂蛋白胆固醇；LDL-C，低密度脂蛋白胆固醇。

表3　心率与血脂、血糖水平的关联

特　征	β	SE	wald	*P*
TC				
Model 1	0.004	0.001	4.01	< 0.01
Model 2	0.003	0.001	2.90	< 0.01

续表

特　征	β	SE	wald	P
TG				
Model 1	0.006	0.001	6.72	< 0.01
Model 2	0.005	0.001	5.71	< 0.01
HDL-C				
Model 1	0.000 2	0.000 4	0.71	> 0.05
Model 2	0.000 1	0.000 3	0.00	> 0.05
LDL-C				
Model 1	0.001 9	0.001 0	1.68	> 0.05
Model 2	0.001 1	0.000 9	1.21	> 0.05
血糖水平				
Model 1	0.010	0.002	6.23	< 0.01
Model 2	0.009	0.002	6.04	< 0.01

Model 1：调整年龄、性别、民族；Model 2：调整 Model 1 + BMI、吸烟、饮酒、教育程度、高血压和居住海拔。

3. 讨论

本研究发现，心率与血脂、血糖水平呈正相关；调整年龄、性别、民族、体重指数、吸烟、饮酒、教育程度、高血压和糖尿病后，该相关性仍具有统计学意义。本次分析未发现心率和居住海拔之间对血脂、血糖的影响存在交互作用。本研究结果提示心率可能作为西藏新疆地区代谢性疾病的预测因子。

与本研究结果类似，澳大利亚一项研究发现男性心率增加可能增加糖尿病的患病风险[10]。美国一项研究同样发现，心率增加可预测糖尿病及相关死亡的发生[9]。国内也有研究发现随着心率的增加高脂血症、高尿酸血症、糖尿病等代谢性疾病的检出率随之增加[11]。最近 Wang 等[7]分析开滦前瞻性队列研究发现静息心率可预测糖尿病的发病风险。

静息心率和血脂异常的研究相对较少，Sun 等[8]在中老年人群中发现心率和血脂异常存在关联。巴西一项前瞻性研究发现静息心率是肥胖青少年人群血脂异常的独立预测因子，而这项研究并未发现静息心率和血糖之间的关联[6]。郭艳英等[12]发现新疆博州地区维、哈、蒙、汉族人群中随着静息心率的增加，肥胖、高血压、高空腹血糖、血脂紊乱等多项心血管病危险因素发生风险增加并发现心率增加容易导致心血管病危险因素聚集出现。之前研究关于静息心率与血脂各个组分关系的结论存在较大争议，如 Sun 等[8]发现高 TC、高 TG、高 LDL-C 随着心率增加患病率逐渐增加，而低 HDL-C 患病率逐渐降低。而本研究仅发现，随着静息心率水平增加，TC、TG 水平和血脂异常的患病率逐渐增加。

静息心率预测血脂异常和糖尿病的机制目前不很明确。研究显示静息心率增加是机体自主神经功能紊乱的表现，心率加快意味着交感神经的激活和副交感神经的抑制[13]。交感神经过度兴奋通过刺激肾上腺素释放引起胰岛素抵抗，增加糖尿病的发病风险[14]。同时通过作用于胰腺、肝脏和骨骼肌，使血糖升高[15]。长期的自主神经系统不平衡增加高血压、动脉粥样硬化的发病风险[16，17]。

本研究首次基于高原地区人群数据分析发现心率与血脂、血糖水平呈正相关，提示心率可能作为心脏代谢性疾病的预测因子，同时本次分析并未发现居住地海拔和心率之间存在交互作用。本研究的优点在于数据来源于大规模且具有代表性的抽样调查，但是由于本次研究并未完全收集到所有血脂异常和糖尿病的危险因素（比如饮食、体力活动等），同时研究本身为横断面设计，故其因果关系需要队列研究进一步验证。

致谢

感谢参与项目的所有专家及所有调查人员。协作组组成单位及主要调查人员：国家心血管病中心、中国医学科学院阜外医院王增武、张林峰、陈祚、王馨、邵澜、郭敏、田野、赵天明、范国辉、董颖、聂静雨、王佳丽、郑聪毅、贾秀云、朱曼璐、王文、陈伟伟、高润霖；卫生部北京医院郭岩斐、孙铁英、王玉霞、柴迪、马雅立、仝亚琪；中国人民解放军总医院陈韵岱、冯斌、朱庆磊、周珊珊、刘杰、王晶、杨丽娜、杨瑛、段鹏；新疆维吾尔自治区人民医院李南方、周玲、张德莲、姚晓光、洪静、索菲亚、曹梅；中国疾病预防控制中心吴静、石文惠、翟屹、何柳。

参考文献

[1] Miller M. Dyslipidemia and cardiovascular risk: the importance of early prevention [J]. QJM, 2009, 102(9): 657-667.

[2] Shah AD, Langenberg C, Rapsomaniki E, et al. Type 2 diabetes and incidence of cardiovascular diseases a cohort study in 1. 9 million people [J]. Lancet Diabetes Endocrinol, 2015, 3(2): 105-113.

[3] Hu SS, Kong LZ, Gao RL, et al. Outline of the report on cardiovascular disease in China, 2010 [J]. Biomed Environ Sci, 2012, 25(3): 251-256.

[4] Grassi G, Vailati S, Bertinieri G, et al. Heart rate as marker of sympathetic activity [J]. J Hypertens, 1998, 16(11): 1635-1639.

[5] Thanou A, Stavrakis S, Dyer JW, et al. Impact of heart rate variability, a marker for cardiac health, on lupus disease activity [J]. Arthritis Res Ther, 2016, 18: 197.

[6] Freitas JI, Monteiro PA, Silveira LS, et al. Resting heart rate as a predictor of metabolic dysfunctions in obese children and adolescents [J]. BMC Pediatr, 2012, 12: 5.

[7] Wang L, Cui L, Wang Y, et al. Resting heart rate and the risk of developing impaired fasting glucose and diabetes the Kailuan prospective study [J]. Int J Epidemiol, 2015, 44(2): 689-699.

[8] Sun JC, Huang XL, Deng XR, et al. Elevated resting heart rate is associated with dyslipidemia in middle-aged and elderly Chinese [J]. Biomed Environ Sci, 2014, 27(8): 601-605.

[9] Shigetoh Y, Adachi H, Yamagishi S, et al. Higher heart rate may predispose to obesity and diabetes mellitus: 20-year prospective study in a general population [J]. Am J Hypertens, 2009, 22(2): 151-155.

[10] Grantham NM, Magliano DJ, Tanamas SK, et al. Higher heart rate increases risk of diabetes among men: The Australian Diabetes Obesity and Lifestyle (AusDiab) Study [J]. Diabet Med, 2013, 30(4): 421-427.

[11] 程敏，张倩，程蓉. 心率与心血管及代谢性疾病的关系分析 [J]. 现代预防医学，2007, 34(11): 2051-2054.

[12] 郭艳英，罗雄，赵蕾，等. 多民族静息心率与心血管危险因素的关系 [J]. 中国医师杂志，2010, 12(3): 318-321.

[13] Robinson BF, Epstein SE, Beiser GD, et al. Control of heart rate by the autonomic nervous system. Studies in man on the interrelation between baroreceptor mechanisms and exercise [J]. Circ Res, 1966, 19(2): 400-411.

[14] Deibert DC, Defronzo RA. Epinephrine-induced insulin resistance in man[J]. J Clin Invest, 1980, 65(3): 717-721.

[15] Shimazu T. Innervation of the liver and glucoregulation: roles of the hypothalamus and autonomic nerves [J]. Nutrition, 1996, 12(1): 65-66.

[16] Yang Z, Xu B, Lu J, et al. Autonomic test by EZSCAN in the screening for prediabetes and diabetes [J]. PLoS One, 2013, 8(2): e56480.

[17] Sun K, Liu Y, Dai M, et al. Accessing autonomic function can early screen metabolic syndrome [J]. PLoS One, 2012, 7(8): e43449.

Prevalence and Risk Factors Associated with Chronic Kidney Disease in Adults Living in 3 Different Altitude Regions in the Tibetan Plateau △

ZHANG Linfeng[1], WANG Zengwu[1,*], CHEN Yundai[2], WANG Xin[1], CHEN Zuo[1], FENG Bin[2], ZHU Qinglei[2], NIE Jingyu[1], DONG Ying[1], ZHOU Shanshan[2], TIAN Ye[1], SHAO Lan[1], ZHU Manlu[1]

1. Division of Prevention and Community Health, National Center for Cardiovascular Disease, Fuwai Hospital, Peking Union Medical College, Chinese Academy of Medical Science, Beijing, China
2. Department of Cardiology, PLA General Hospital, Beijing 100853, China

Abstract **Background** Living at high altitude may have undesirable effects on the kidney. We explored the chronic kidney disease(CKD) prevalence and risk factors among the residents living at different altitude in Tibetan Plateau. **Methods** A cross-sectional study was carried out in 2014 to 2016 in Linzhi(2 900 m altitude), Lhasa(3 650 m)and Anduo(4 700 m). Information on the cardiovascular risk factors was collected and blood and urine samples were measured. **Results** The data of 1 707 subjects aged ≥ 35 y were analyzed. The age-standardized prevalence of CKD in Linzhi, Lhasa and Anduo was 27.7%(95% CI: 22.1–33.3%), 18.3%(12.7–24.0%) and 30.4%(23.5–37.3%) in men and 37.7%(31.8–43.6%), 29.5%(24.6–34.4%) and 36.7%(29.0–44.4%) in women, respectively. multivariatle logistic regression showed that age, female gender, systolic blood pressure, fasting serum glucose, with primary school education or lower were associated with higher risk of CKD and living in Lhasa was associated with lower risk of CKD. **Conclusions** A higher prevalence of CKD was found in the residents living in the Tibetan Plateau. However, for the highlanders living at higher altitude does not mean higher risk. The CKD risk factors found in this study are similar to those in other studies

Keywords Chronic kidney disease; Prevalence; Epidemiology; Tibet; High altitude

1. Background

Chronic kidney disease(CKD) can not only lead to end-stage renal disease, dialysis and

△ 本文发表于：Clinica Chimica Acta, 2018, 481: 212-217.

transplantation therapy, but also plays an important role in drug toxicity, endocrine and metabolic outcomes, and cardiovascular disease [1-5]. Early detection and intervention can prevent or delay complications of decreased kidney function, slow the progression of kidney disease and reduce the risk of cardiovascular disease(CVD) [6]. Therefore, it is necessary to carry out studies on the prevalence and related risk factors of CKD in order to develop public health policies and strategies to improve the outcomes.

More than140 million people in the world currently live at high altitude(> 2 400 m) [7]. As the altitude increases, the concentration of oxygen in the air decreases rapidly. It is estimated that at 4 000 m, every lungful of air only has 60% of the oxygen molecules that people at sea level have [8]. Living at high altitude under hypoxic conditions may have undesirable effects on the kidney [9, 10]. Is living at high altitude a major risk factor for CKD among the highland residents? Although a study conducted by Chen et al[11]. in the Tibetan population living in Lhasa city and Dangxiong County found a higher prevalence of CKD compared with that in Guangzhou and Beijing, the high-altitude, mountainous and harsh geographical features make the way of life of the people living in Tibet markedly different from the east of China. On the other hand, data show that the highlanders exhibit unique "hypoxiatolerant" physiological characteristics, especially among the Tibetan ethnicity [12]. To answer this question, it is better to conduct a study among the populations living at different altitude and with similar genetic background and way of life.

Tibetan Plateau is one of the highest areas with people living on Earth, with an average elevation of 4 900 m and most of the residents are Tibetan ethnicity. Although numerous studies have reported the prevalence of chronic kidney disease(CKD) [11, 13-19], the data on people living in different altitude regions in the Tibetan Plateau are sparse. In this study, we explored the prevalence of CKD and its associations with cardiovascular disease(CVD) risk factors among the residents living at an altitude of 2 900 m, 3 650 m and 4 700 m in the Tibetan Plateau.

2. Methods

2.1 Study design and participants

A cross-sectional survey on cardiovascular disease and related risk factors was conducted in Linzhi County(abbreviated as Linzhi, with an altitude of 2 900 m above sea level), Chengguan district in Lhasa city(Lhasa, altitude 3 650 m) and Anduo County(Anduo, altitude 4 700 m)in the Tibet Autonomous Region in China from the year of 2014 to 2016. The participants were selected from each county or district with a multistage random sampling method. First, 2 towns(or street offices) were selected from each county(or district); second, three villages or communities were selected from each town(or street offices); finally all the residents who were ≥ 15 y and living in the villages or communities for more than half a year were stratified by sex and age and randomly sampled from each sex and age group. Simple random sampling method was used in each stage. Due to the harsh environment, small population size and large geographic span, only one town was selected in Anduo County. In Linzhi, Lhasa and Anduo, 1 563, 1 120 and 1 600 residents were invited to participate in the study, and 1 080, 1 108 and 1 029 residents were enrolled and completed the survey and examination, respectively. Written informed consent was obtained from all participants and institutional review board approval was obtained from the Fuwai Hospital.

For the participants < 35 y, due to the low compliance to blood drawing, blood and urine samples were not collected. Moreover, for this analysis, we excluded those participants with missing data for the variables analyzed. Therefore, only the data of the participants aged ≥ 35 y and with complete data were analyzed in this study(Fig.1). In detail, we excluded 1 262 participants with age < 35 and 113 individuals without serum creatinine, urinary albumin or creatinine test results. Of the 1 762 participants, we further excluded 2 individuals without total cholesterol(TC) and other blood chemistry test results, 10 individuals without systolic or diastolic blood pressure values and 43 individuals without smoking and other lifestyle information. The final sample for analysis comprised 1 707 participants.

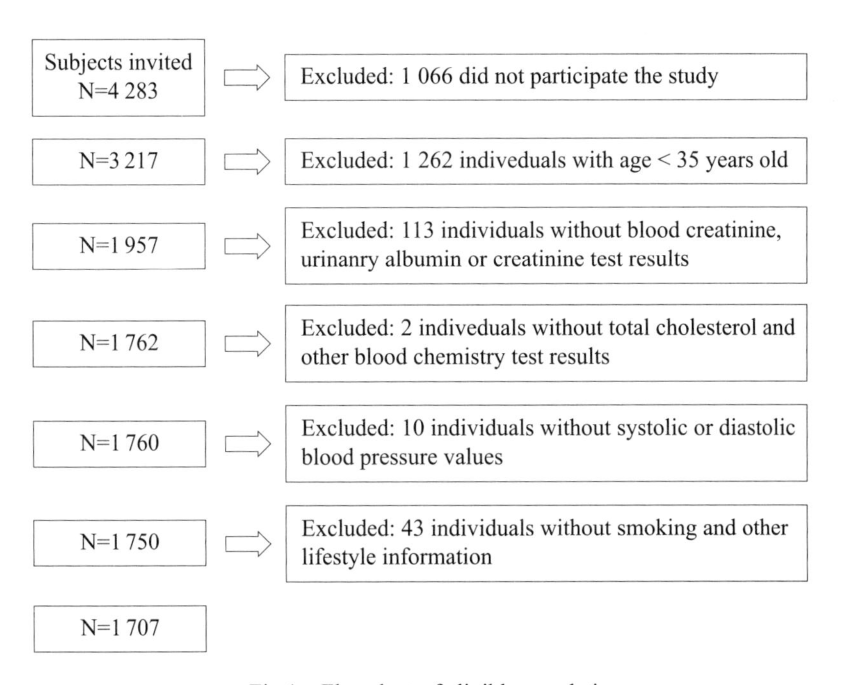

Fig.1 Flowchart of eligible population.

2.2 Data collection and measurements

The demographic, personal habits such as smoking and alcohol consumption, personal and family history of cardiovascular disease, and physical examination data were collected by trained research staff per the study protocol. Smoking status was classified into 2 categories: current smokers and non-smokers. Alcohol consumption was classified into 2 categories: current drinkers and non-drinkers. Height was measured in standing position without shoes, using a standard stadiometer. Body weight was measured with light clothing. Waist circumference was measured midway between the bottom edge of the last rib and iliac crest in the mid-axillary plane using a cloth tape directly touching the participant's skin. Systolic blood pressure(SBP) and diastolic blood pressure(DBP) were measured 3 times with the participant in sitting position using digital blood pressure monitor(OMRON HBP1 300). The participant was asked to sit quietly and rest for at least 5 min with his/her legs uncrossed and an empty bladder. Three blood pressure measurements were taken and the participants rested at least 1 min between each of the readings. If 2 readings differed by > 10 mmHg, remeasurement was done. The average of the 3 measurements was used for analysis. BMI was calculated using the formula weight/height^2(kg/m^2). If a subject's parents or siblings have been reported to have the history of hypertension, diabetes mellitus, stroke and coronary heart disease, the subject was considered to have family history of cardiovascular disease(CVD).

All blood samples were obtained in the morning after at least 8-h overnight fast, and biochemical assays were performed at a central laboratory. The serum glucose was determined using enzymatic method. Serum TC, triglyceride(TG) were determined using enzymatic methods, low-density lipoprotein cholesterol(LDL-C), high-density lipoprotein cholesterol(HDL-C) were determined using direct assay with an autoanalyzer(Beckman AU400), and LDL-C was calculated with Friedewald formula when TG < 4.52 mmol/l. Urinary albumin was measured using turbidimetric inhibition immunoassay. Urinary creatinine and serum creatinine were measured by Jaffe's kinetic method. Urinary albumin to creatinine ratio(ACR) was calculated. The estimated glomerular filtration rate(eGFR) was calculated using the CKD-EPI equation [20]. The eGFR was categorized as: normal or high(≥ 90 ml/min/1.73 m^2), mildly decreased(60 – 89 ml/min/1.73 m^2) and moderately to severely decreased(< 60 ml/min/1.73 m^2). The albuminuria was categorized as: normal to mildly increased(ACR < 30 mg/g), moderately increased(ACR 30 mg/g to < 300 mg/g) and severely increased(ACR ≥ 300 mg/g). CKD was defined as either decreased eGFR(eGFR < 60 ml/min/1.73 m^2) or albuminuria(ACR ≥ 30 mg/g) according to Kidney Disease Improving Global Outcomes(KDIGO)guidelines [21].

2.3 Statistical analysis

Data for continuous variables were presented as mean ± SD and tested for normality with the Shapiro-Wilk test, then compared with analysis of variance(ANOVA) or Kruskal-Wallis test where appropriate; Data for categorical variables were presented as count and proportions and compared with χ^2 test. The prevalence of CKD was presented for different age groups, genders and regions. Age standardization was performed with the China 2 010 Census population. Cochran-Armitage trend test was used to determine if age was correlated with the prevalence of CKD. To explore the factors associated with CKD, univariable logistic regression analysis was performed first, then for the factors which has a $P < 0.1$ stepwise binary logistic regression analysis with stepwise method was performed to explore the influencing factors. The significant levels for a variable to enter into or stay in the model were both 0.05. Unless stated otherwise, all P values were 2 sided and $P < 0.05$ were considered statistically significant. The analyses were carried out using SAS ver. 9.4.

Table 1 Characteristics of the study participants

Parameters	Men				Women			
	Linzhi(n = 275)	Lhasa(n = 197)	Anduo(n = 232)	P-value	Linzhi(n = 341)	Lhasa(n = 419)	Anduo(n = 243)	P-value
Age (y)	51.2 ± 11.9	53.1 ± 10.9	48.2 ± 10.6	< 0.001	51.5 ± 11.1	53.3 ± 10.5	47.8 ± 10.1	< 0.001
Tibetan ethinic, n(%)	219(79.6)	173(87.8)	225(97.0)	< 0.001	323(94.7)	389(92.8)	238(97.9)	0.018
BMI (kg/m^2)	24.7 ± 3.6	25.7 ± 3.4	25.8 ± 4.0	0.001	24.7 ± 3.7	26.5 ± 4.1	26.8 ± 4.5	< 0.001
WC (cm)	88.3 ± 11.1	89.5 ± 8.9	88.9 ± 10.6	NS	81.2 ± 12.0	89.8 ± 11.2	86.7 ± 12.2	< 0.001
SBP (mmHg)	134.6 ± 22.1	137.2 ± 21.5	124.6 ± 20.1	< 0.001	132.1 ± 22.8	135.0 ± 21.9	120.4 ± 21.9	< 0.001
DBP (mmHg)	85.5 ± 13.7	85.4 ± 12.4	80.4 ± 14.6	< 0.001	81.3 ± 12.6	81.9 ± 13.2	76.4 ± 13.9	< 0.001
TC (mmol/l)	4.65 ± 0.93	4.78 ± 1.01	4.59 ± 0.95	NS	4.53 ± 0.89	4.98 ± 0.94	4.28 ± 0.89	< 0.001
LDL-C (mmol/l)	2.68 ± 0.80	2.83 ± 0.85	2.91 ± 0.87	0.007	2.56 ± 0.75	2.90 ± 0.77	2.55 ± 0.74	< 0.001
HDL-C (mmol/l)	1.42 ± 0.33	1.40 ± 0.33	1.21 ± 0.26	< 0.001	1.57 ± 0.29	1.61 ± 0.36	1.36 ± 0.30	< 0.001
TG (mmol/l)	1.26 ± 1.02	1.24 ± 0.79	1.03 ± 0.59	0.003	0.88 ± 0.45	1.04 ± 0.55	0.80 ± 0.37	< 0.001
Fasting blood glucose (mmol/l)	5.35 ± 2.57	4.54 ± 1.47	4.94 ± 1.26	< 0.001	4.73 ± 0.83	4.37 ± 1.43	4.79 ± 1.51	< 0.001
Current smoker, n(%)	98(35.6)	79(40.1)	81(34.9)	NS	6(1.8)	6(1.4)	16(6.6)	< 0.001
Current drinker, n(%)	34(12.4)	40(20.3)	8(3.4)	< 0.001	3(0.9)	2(0.5)	0(0.0)	NS
Primary school education or lower, n(%)	187(68.0)	149(75.6)	175(75.4)	NS	307(90.0)	350(83.5)	200(82.3)	0.012

续表

Parameters	Men				Women			
	Linzhi(n = 275)	Lhasa(n = 197)	Anduo(n = 232)	P-value	Linzhi(n = 341)	Lhasa(n = 419)	Anduo(n = 243)	P-value
eGFR (ml/min per 1.73 m2)	89.7 ± 13.7	88.4 ± 12.4	87.8 ± 13.1	NS	89.4 ± 14.3	84.2 ± 13.8	86.9 ± 14.0	< 0.001
ACR (mg/g)	63.4 ± 325.5	31.3 ± 84.9	117.7 ± 486.1	NS	46.2 ± 221.1	33.9 ± 60.1	100.0 ± 478.1	0.010
History of CHD or stroke, n(%)	0(0.0)	1(0.5)	3(1.3)	NS	0(0.0)	10(2.4)	2(0.8)	0.009
Family history of CVD, n(%)	91(33.1)	75(38.1)	83(35.8)	NS	106(31.1)	161(38.4)	122(50.2)	< 0.001

Data are means ± SD or number of participants(%). Abbreviations: WC, waist circumference; SBP, systolic blood pressure; DBP, diastolic blood pressure; ACR, albumin to creatinine ratio. The data were compared with analysis of variance(ANOVA) or Kruskal-Wallis test for continuous variables and χ^2 test for categorical variables.

3. Results

3.1 Demographic and clinical data of the subjects analyzed

Table 1 summarized the characteristics of the participants in Linzhi, Lhasa and Anduo. In men, there is no difference among the 3 regions for WC, TC, eGFR, ACR and the proportion of the subjects with smoking, primary school education or lower, history of CHD or stroke and family history of CVD. In women, except the proportion of current drinkers, all the other characteristics differed significantly among the 3 regions. In both men and women, the participants living in Anduo tended to be younger and more Tibetan ethnic and had lower SBP, DBP, HDL-C and TG levels than the other 2 regions.

3.2 Prevalence of the chronic kidney disease

Table 2 shows the proportions of the participants in each eGFR or albuminuria category and CKD prevalence for both men and women in each region. The proportions of the participants with eGFR < 60 ml/min per 1.73 m^2 were all very small for each region and most cases of CKD were diagnosed with moderate or severe albuminuria. The prevalence of CKD in Linzhi, Lhasa and Anduo was 27.6%, 19.3% and 25.4% in men and 37.0%, 30.3% and 30.4% in women, respectively. The older participants had a higher prevalence of CKD in all 3 regions(Fig.2). Except the ≥ 65 year age group of the women for all other age groups the prevalence of CKD in Linzhi is higher than that in Lasha in both men and women, but only the difference in the 55 – 64 age group among men was of statistical significance(P = 0.006). The age-standardized prevalence of CKD in Linzhi, Lhasa and Anduo was 27.7%(95 confidence interval 22.1–33.3%), 18.3%(12.7–24.0%) and 30.4%(23.5–37.3%) in men and 37.7%(31.8–43.6%), 29.5%(24.6–34.4%) and 36.7%(29.0–44.4%) in women, respectively. If the 57 subjects with incomplete data were included, the prevalence of CKD in Linzhi, Lhasa and Anduo was 27.5%, 19.4% and 25.9% in men and 37.0%, 29.7% and 30.8% in women, respectively. The CKD prevalence in Lhasa was still lower than that in Linzhi in both men and women($P = 0.038$ in men and $P = 0.033$ in women, respectively).

Table 2 Prevalence of chronic kidney disease(CKD) by gender and region

Sex/area	n	eGFR (ml/min per 1.73 m^2)			ACR (mg/g)			CKD
		≥ 90	60 – 89	< 60	< 30	30 – 299	≥ 300	
Men								
Linzhi	275	143(52.0)[a]	128(46.5)	4(1.5)	200(72.7)	68(24.7)	7(2.6)	76(27.6)
Lhasa	197	85(43.2)	110(55.8)	2(1.0)	161(81.7)	34(17.3)	2(1.0)	38(19.3)
Anduo	232	108(46.5)	119(51.3)	5(2.2)	174(75.3)	46(19.8)	12(5.2)	59(25.4)
Women								
Linzhi	341	180(52.8)	145(42.5)	16(4.7)	222(65.1)	117(34.3)	2(0.6)	126(37.0)
Lhasa	419	139(33.2)	257(61.3)	23(5.5)	306(73.0)	108(25.8)	5(1.2)	127(30.3)
Anduo	243	92(37.9)	143(58.8)	8(3.3)	173(71.2)	61(25.1)	9(3.7)	73(30.4)

[a] Data are number of participants(%). Abbreviations: eGFR, estimated glomerular filtration rate; ACR, albumin to creatinine ratio; CKD, chronic kidney disease. CKD was defined as eGFR < 60 ml/min/1.73 m^2 and/or ACR ≥ 30 mg/g.

3.3 Risk factors associated with CKD

Before conducting multivariable stepwise logistic regression analysis, univariable analysis of the associations between the risk factors and CKD was performed first(Table 3). The results demonstrated that region, age, gender, Tibetan ethnicity, BMI, SBP, DBP, TC, HDL-C, GLU, smoking, drinking, education level and with history of CHD or stroke were the major factors associated with CKD and had $P < 0.1$.

Table 3 Univariable logistic regression analysis of the factors associated with CKD

Parameters	Regression coefficient	SE	Wald	*P*	OR(95% CI)
Region[a]					
Linzhi(reference)	—	—	—	—	1.00
Lhasa	- 0.287 9	0.125 1	5.299 3	0.021	0.750(0.587 - 0.958)
Anduo	- 0.237 3	0.133 6	3.154 4	0.076	0.789(0.607 - 1.025)
Age(years)	0.045 5	0.004 93	85.135 7	< 0.001	1.047(1.036 - 1.057)
Female	0.390 7	0.110 5	12.501 4	< 0.001	1.478(1.190 - 1.835)
Tibetan ethinic	0.853 2	0.238 6	12.784 3	< 0.001	2.347(1.470 - 3.747)
BMI(kg/m^2)	0.024 4	0.013 4	3.344 9	0.067	1.025(0.998 - 1.052)
WC(cm)	0.003 24	0.004 59	0.498 5	0.480	1.003(0.994 - 1.012)
SBP(mmHg)	0.028 5	0.002 50	130.265 1	< 0.001	1.029(1.024 - 1.034)
DBP(mmHg)	0.037 4	0.004 04	85.756 8	< 0.001	1.038(1.030 - 1.046)
TC(mmol/L)	0.139 0	0.055 2	6.344 2	0.012	1.149(1.031 - 1.280)
LDL-C(mmol/L)	0.099 4	0.065 6	2.296 0	0.130	1.105(0.971 - 1.256)
HDL-C(mmol/L)	0.401 8	0.152 7	6.920 4	0.009	1.495(1.108 - 2.016)
TG(mmol/L)	0.086 0	0.077 1	1.244 5	0.265	1.090(0.937 - 1.268)
GLU(mmol/L)	0.095 7	0.031 9	9.012 2	0.008	1.100(1.034 - 1.171)
Current smoker	- 0.521 1	0.156 2	11.134 5	< 0.001	0.594(0.437 - 0.807)
Current drinker	- 0.634 0	0.282 0	5.053 2	0.025	0.530(0.305 - 0.922)
Primary school education or lower	0.908 7	0.158 2	32.983 4	< 0.001	2.481(1.820 - 3.383)
History of CHD or stroke	0.893 3	0.502 9	3.156 0	0.076	2.443(0.912 - 6.547)
Family history of CVD	- 0.018 2	0.110 1	0.027 3	0.869	0.982(0.791 - 1.218)

Abbreviations: CKD, chronic kidney disease; BMI, Body mass index; WC, waist circumference; SBP, systolic blood pressure; DBP, diastolic blood pressure; TC, total cholesterol; LDL-C, low-density lipoprotein cholesterol; HDL-C, high-density lipoprotein cholesterol; TG, triglycerides; GLU, fasting blood glucose; CHD, coronary heart disease; CVD, cardiovascular disease; SE, standard error; OR, odds ratio; CI, confidence interval.

[a] The reference category is Linzhi.

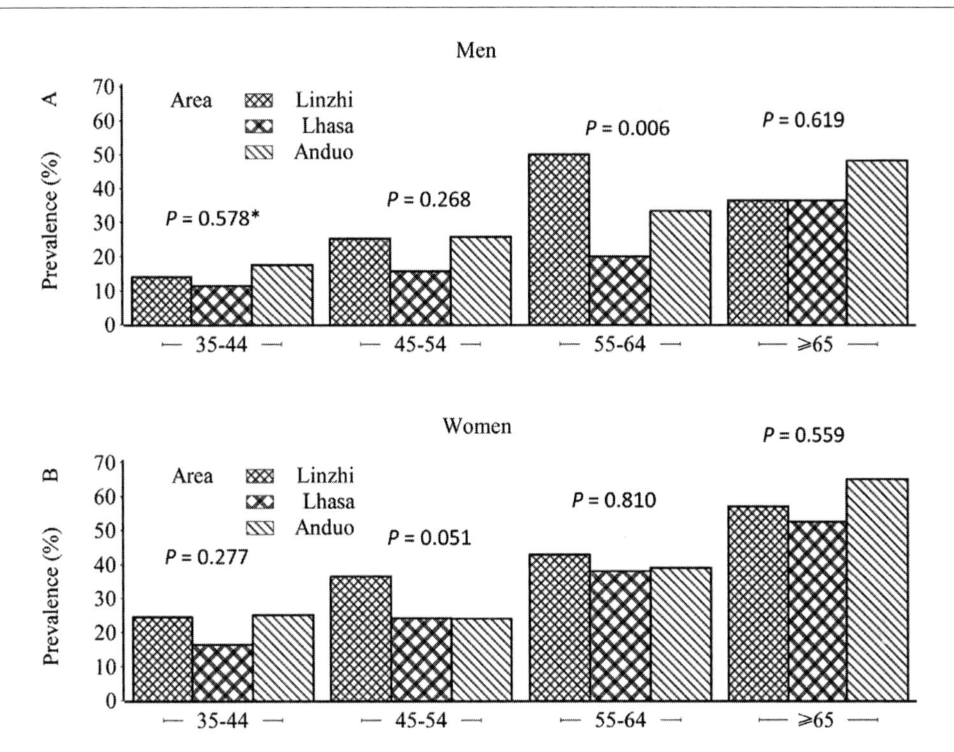

Fig.2 A and B, prevalence of chronic kidney disease(CKD) by age and sex in Linzhi, Lhasa and Anduo. The prevalence of CKD was 14.0%, 25.3%, 50.0%, and 36.4% in Linzhi, 11.4%, 15.7%, 20.0%, and 36.4% in Lhasa, and 17.6%, 25.7%, 33.3%, and 48.1% in Anduo in the age range 35-44, 45-54, 55-64 and 65 years and over in men(A); 24.5%, 36.4%, 42.9%, and 56.9% in Linzhi, 16.3%, 24.1%, 37.9%, and 52.5% in Lhasa, 25.0%, 24.0%, 38.9%, and 65.0% in Anduo in the age range 35-44, 45-54, 55-64 and 65 years and over in women (B). *P* for trend was < 0.001 in all three regions in both genders(Tested with Cochran-Armitage trend test). *, *P* value for the chi-square test of the difference of CKD prevalence among the three regions in each gender and age group.

Therefore, these factors were analyzed with a stepwise logistic regression analysis(Table 4). The results showed that age, female gender, higher level of SBP, GLU, with primary school education or lower, and living in Lhasa were independently associated with the occurrence of CKD($P < 0.05$, respectively).

Table 4 Stepwise logistic regression analysis of the factors associated with CKD

Parameters	Regression coefficient	SE	Wald	*P*	OR(95% CI)
Intercept	− 6.588 5	0.468 7	197.576 2	< 0.000 1	—
Areaa					
Linzhi (reference)	—	—	—	—	1.00

续表

Parameters	Regression coefficient	SE	Wald	*P*	OR(95% CI)
Lhasa	− 0.467 0	0.139 3	11.240 0	< 0.001	0.627(0.477 − 0.824)
Anduo	0.122 4	0.148 3	0.681 4	0.409	1.130(0.845 − 1.511)
Age (years)	0.019 9	0.006 05	10.883 0	0.001	1.020(1.008 − 1.032)
Female	0.531 3	0.123 8	18.433 5	< 0.001	1.701(1.335 − 2.168)
SBP (mmHg)	0.027 1	0.002 94	85.234 6	< 0.001	1.028(1.022 − 1.033)
GLU (mmol/L)	0.093 1	0.034 0	7.485 8	0.006	1.098(1.027 − 1.173)
Primary school education or lower	0.479 4	0.171 4	7.817 7	0.005	1.615(1.154 − 2.260)

Abbreviations: CKD, chronic kidney disease; SBP, systolic blood pressure; GLU, fasting blood glucose; SE, standard error; OR, odds ratio; CI, confidence interval.

[a] The reference category is Linzhi.

4. Discussion

In this study that conducted in the residents living in 3 regions with different altitude in the Tibetan Plateau, we did not detect systematic differences in prevalence of CKD according to altitude. On the contrary, our data showed that compared with the residents living in Linzhi with an altitude of 2 900 m, living at Lhasa(altitude 3 650 m) was associated with lower risk for CKD. Multivariable logistic regression analysis showed that the independent risk factors associated with CKD among the highlanders included age, female gender, systolic blood pressure, fasting serum glucose, with primary school education or lower, and living in Lhasa was a protective factor.

It is believed that living at high altitude under hypoxic condition has many effects on the kidney and may cause high altitude renal syndrome [9, 10]. However, in contrast to the notion that living at higher altitude will have higher risk of CKD, the multivariable logistic regression analysis showed that the residents living in Lhasa had a 25% lower risk of CKD than those in Linzhi and there was no significant difference for the risk of CKD between Anduo and Linzhi. The probable explanation for this phenomenon may be that Tibetan highlanders may have evolved to adapt the high-altitude environment [12, 22] and altitude is not the major determinant of the risk of CKD among the highland residents, other factors may be more important. Many factors such as age, gender, hypertension and diabetes have been reported to be related to CKD [14, 19, 23]. In our study, SBP was shown to be a risk factor of CKD in the multivariate logistic analysis and the residents living in

Anduo have the lowest level of SBP in both men and women(Table 1). Other factors associated with CKD in the multivariable logistic analysis in this study included age, female gender, fasting serum glucose, and with primary school education or lower. On the other hand, our study did show a higher prevalence of CKD in the Tibetan population as that in the previous reports. The study conducted by Chen et al. [11] in the Tibet population living in Lhasa city and Dangxiong County found a higher prevalence of CKD compared with that in Guangzhou and Beijing. In our study, we included the residents living in Lhasa, too. The age-standardized prevalence of CKD in Lhasa was 18.8% in men and 30.1% in women, in contrast with 18.9% in men and 19.9% in women in Chen's study. The prevalence of CKD in women in our study is higher than that Chen's study, which may be partially explained by the fact that we included older subjects in our study. In our study we only enrolled the subjects aged ⩾ 35 y, while in Chen's study they enrolled subjects aged ⩾ 18 y. Other explanation may include different GFR estimation equation used, different laboratory conditions and reagents and sampling errors. The prevalence of CKD in the general adult populations is reported to be 10–17% in the USA [13], Norway [15], and Australia [17]. The prevalence of CKD in the Chinese general populations was reported to be 10.8% in a national survey [14], and other studies reported a lower CKD prevalence [18, 19]. However, the mean ages of the study populations are different. In Zhang's study they also reported the prevalence of CKD in different age groups in the supplemental data [14]. The prevalence of CKD in Zhang's study in the age group 18–39, 40–59, 60–69 and ⩾ 70 years was 5.1%, 8.3%, 13.2%, 18.5% in men and 7.4%, 11.9%, 18.0%, 24.2% in women, respectively. Although the cut-off points of the age group in our study are different from that in Zhang's study(Fig.2), we can deduce the prevalence of CKD in the Tibetan population is higher. Given the large difference of lifestyle and risk factor profiles between the residents living in Tibetan plateau and the other parts of China [24], whether the factors other than altitude play a more important role in the difference of CKD prevalence between the residents living in Tibetan plateau and other parts of China needs to be further investigated.

The factors related to CKD found in this study are similar to those reported in the previous studies. Older age, being female, hypertension, high fasting glucose have been reported in other studies [14, 19, 23, 25]. In this study, we only explored the association of major CVD risk factors with CKD, there are many other factors we did not explore. For example, in some studies low socioeconomic status has been associated with an increased risk of CKD [26, 27]. Lhasa is the capital of Tibet autonomous region, the quality of health care is better and the residents have more health knowledge than in other regions, which may be one of the possible explanations of the phenomenon that residents living in Lhasa was associated with lower risk of CKD.

Our results have important public health implications for the prevention of CKD in highland residents. To our knowledge, it is the first study to explore the influence of altitude on the prevalence of CKD among the populations living at different altitude in the Tibetan plateau. Our study showed that living at high altitude did not mean a higher risk of CKD among the highlanders, the major risk factors of CKD in the highlanders were similar to that in other regions. Therefore, it is as important for the highlanders to control the known risk factors of CKD as in other regions. On the other hand, studies have shown Tibetans are adapted well to the hypoxic environment, they exhibit distinctive physiological traits and to be resistant to certain pathophysiological processes, such as the maintaining a high resting ventilation and brisk hypoxic ventilatory sensitivities [28, 29], blunted erythropoietic response to hypoxia [30], remarkably low prevalence of chronic mountain sickness [31], protection against the occurrence of intrauterine growth restriction(IUGR) [32], whether the distinctive oxygen-transport traits found in Tibetans can protect them from CKD is unknown. It is the first time for us to find that altitude is not a major risk factor for CKD among the highlanders living in the Tibetan plateau. However, given the higher CKD prevalence in the residents living in Tibetan plateau compared with the other regions in China, it is also important to clarify the underlying mechanism to better control of CKD.

This study had some limitations. Firstly, the cross-sectional design of the study limits the causal inference ability of the study, therefore further studies are needed to verify the findings. Secondly, CKD is usually defined as either decreased eGFR(eGFR < 60 ml/min/1.73 m^2 or albuminuria(ACR $\geqslant 30$ mg/g) longer than 3 months. In this study there was only one blood and urine sample obtained from each participant, which made it impossible to confirm whether the low eGFR or albuminuria were persistent and might have led to an overestimation of CKD. Thirdly, the blood and urine samples were transported to the central lab to determine the level of the serum cholesterol, blood glucose, creatinine, urine albumin and creatinine, the influence of the transport and storage should be assessed. Fourthly, only the major CVD risk factors were explored in this study, to better understand the mechanisms underlying the phenomenon, other factors such as hemoglobin, uric acid, hematocrit should be added to the study. Fifthly, we did not include the subjects who is < 35 years old in our analysis, for such subjects, further studies are needed.

5. Conclusions

In summary, although the prevalence of CKD in the Tibet populations is higher, among the residents living in Tibetan Plateau, higher altitude does not mean a higher risk of CKD among the subjects aged 35 years and above. We found some CVD risk factors were independently related to the risk of CKD, while most of them have been reported in other studies. More investigation are needed to clarify the causal factors for CKD in subjects living at high altitude.

Acknowledgements

The authors acknowledge the contributions of the principal investigators and subcenters. The principal investigators and subcenters are as follows: Cardiovascular Institute and Fu Wai Hospital: Zengwu Wang, Linfeng Zhang, Xin Wang, Zuo Chen, Lan Shao, Min Guo, Ye Tian, Tianming Zhao, Guohui Fan, Ying Dong, Jingyu Nie, Jiali Wang, Congyi Zheng, Xiuyun Jia, Manlu Zhu, Wen Wang, Weiwei Chen, Runlin Gao; Beijing Hospital, National Center of Gerontology: Yanfei Guo, Yuxia Wang, Yaqi Tong; Yali Ma, Di Chai, Tieying Sun; General Hospital of the Chinese Peoploe's Liberation Army: Yundai Chen, Bin Feng, Qinglei Zhu, Shanshan Zhou, Jie Liu, Jing Wang, Lina Yang, Ying Yang, Peng Duan; Jiaxuan Wang; Renmin Hospital of the Xinjiang Uygur Autonomous Region: Nanfang Li, Ling Zhou, Delian Zhang, Xiaoguang Yao, Jing Hong, Suofeiya, Mei Cao; Chinese Center for Disease Control and Prevention: Jing Wu, Yi Zhai, Wenhui Shi, Fang Liu, Liu He.

Funding

This work was supported by the National Health and Family Planning Commission of the Peoples' Republic of China(200902001, 201402002). The authors have also received support from Omron Corporation, Kyoto, Japan, for body fat and weight measurement(Vbody HBF-359).

References

[1] B. K. Mahmoodi, K. Matsushita, M. Woodward, et al., Associations of kidney disease measures with mortality and end-stage renal disease in individuals with and without hypertension: a meta-analysis, Lancet 380(2012) 1649-1661.

[2] C. S. Fox, K. Matsushita, M. Woodward, H. J. Bilo, et al., Associations of kidney disease measures with mortality and end-stage renal disease in individuals with and without diabetes: a meta-analysis, Lancet 380(2012) 1662-1673.

[3] A. Roggeri, D. P. Roggeri, C. Zocchetti, et al., Healthcare costs of the progression of chronic kidney disease and different dialysis techniques estimated through administrative database analysis, J. Nephrol.30(2017) 263-269.

[4] M. Rigoni, E. Torri, G. Nollo, D. Zarantonello, A. Laudon, L. Sottini, G. M. Guarrera, G. Brunori, Survival and time-to-transplantation of peritoneal dialysis versus hemodialysis for end-stage renal disease patients:

competing-risks regression model in a single Italian center experience, J. Nephrol.30(2017) 441-447.

[5] M. Liu, X. C. Li, L. Lu, et al., Cardiovascular disease and its relationship with chronic kidney disease, Eur. Rev. Med. Pharmacol. Sci.18(2014) 2918-2926.

[6] A. S. Levey, S. P. Andreoli, T. DuBose, et al., Chronic kidney disease: common, harmful and treatable-World Kidney Day 2007, Am. J. Kidney Dis.49(2007)175-179.

[7] L. G. Moore, Human genetic adaptation to high altitude, High Alt. Med. Biol.2(2001) 257-279.

[8] T. Hornbein, R. Schoene, High Altitude: An Exploration of Human Adaptation(Lung Biology in Health and Disease), Marcel Dekker, New York, USA, 2001, pp.42-874.

[9] A. M. Luks, R. J. Johnson, E. R. Swenson, Chronic kidney disease at high altitude, J. Am. Soc. Nephrol.19(2008) 2262-2271.

[10] A. H. Arestegui, R. Fuquay, J. Sirota, et al., High altitude renal syndrome(HARS), J. Am. Soc. Nephrol. 22(2011) 1963-1968.

[11] W. Chen, Q. Liu, H. Wang, et al., Prevalence and risk factors of chronic kidney disease: a population study in the Tibetan population, Nephrol. Dial. Transplant.26 (2011) 1592-1599.

[12] R. L. Ge, T. S. Simonson, V. Gordeuk, et al., Metabolic aspects of high-altitude adaptation in Tibetans, Exp. Physiol.100(2015) 1247-1255.

[13] D. Murphy, C. E. McCulloch, F. Lin, et al., Trends in prevalence of chronic kidney disease in the United States, Ann. Intern. Med.165(2016) 473-481.

[14] L. Zhang, F. Wang, L. Wang, et al., Prevalence of chronic kidney disease in China: a cross-sectional survey, Lancet 379(2012) 815-822.

[15] S. I. Hallan, J. Coresh, B. C. Astor, et al., International comparison of the relationship of chronic kidney disease prevalence and ESRD risk, J. Am. Soc. Nephrol.17(2006)2275-2284.

[16] C. G. Okwuonu, I. I. Chukwuonye, O. A. Adejumo, et al., Prevalence of chronic kidney disease and its risk factors among adults in a semi-urban community of South-East Nigeria, Niger. Postgrad. Med. J.24(2017) 81-87.

[17] S. J. Chadban, E. M. Briganti, P. G. Kerr, et al., Prevalence of kidney damage in Australian adults: the AusDiab kidney study, J. Am. Soc. Nephrol.14(Suppl.2) (2003) S131-138.

[18] L. Xue, Y. Lou, X. Feng, et al., Prevalence of chronic kidney disease and associated factors among the Chinese population in Taian, China, BMC Nephrol.15(2014) 205.

[19] L. Pan, R. Ma, Y. Wu, et al., Prevalence and risk factors associated with chronic kidney disease in a Zhuang ethnic minority area in China, Nephrology(Carlton) 20 (2015) 807-813.

[20] A. S. Levey, L. A. Stevens, C. H. Schmid, et al., CKD-EPI(chronic kidney disease epidemiology collaboration). A new equation to estimate glomerular filtration rate, Ann. Intern. Med.150(2009) 604-612.

[21] P. E. Stevens, A. Levin, Kidney Disease: Improving Global Outcomes Chronic Kidney Disease Guideline

Development Work Group Members. Evaluation and management of chronic kidney disease: synopsis of the kidney disease: improving global outcomes 2012 clinical practice guideline, Ann. Intern. Med.158(2013) 825-830.

[22] C. M. Beall, G. L. Cavalleri, L. Deng, et al., Natural selection on EPAS1(HIF2alpha) associated with low hemoglobin concentration in Tibetan highlanders, Proc. Natl. Acad. Sci. U. S. A.107(2010) 11459-11464.

[23] W. Chen, W. Chen, H. Wang, et al., Prevalence and risk factors associated with chronic kidney disease in an adult population from southern China, Nephrol. Dial. Transplant.24(2009) 1205-1212.

[24] Y. S. Hu, C. H. Yao, W. Z. Wang, et al., Survey on the prevalence of hypertension in different ethnic groups in China in 2002, Wei Sheng Yan Jiu 35(2006) 573-575(in Chinese).

[25] Z. Y. Li, G. B. Xu, T. A. Xia, et al., Prevalence of chronic kidney disease in a middle and old-aged population of Beijing, Clin. Chim. Acta 366(2006) 209-215.

[26] C. M. Fored, E. Ejerblad, J. P. Fryzek, et al., Socio-economic status and chronic renal failure: a population-based case-control study in Sweden, Nephrol. Dial. Transplant.18(2003) 82-88.

[27] S. S. Merkin, A. V. Diez Roux, J. Coresh, et al., Individual and neighborhood socioeconomic status and progressive chronic kidney disease in an elderly population: The Cardiovascular Health Study, Soc. Sci. Med.65(2007) 809-821.

[28] P. H. Hackett, J. T. Reeves, C. D. Reeves, et al., Control of breathing in Sherpas at low and high altitude, J. Appl. Physiol. Respir. Environ. Exerc. Physiol.49(1980)374-379.

[29] J. Zhuang, T. Droma, S. Sun, et al., Hypoxic ventilatory responsiveness in Tibetan compared with Han residents of 3, 658 m, J. Appl. Physiol.74(1993) 303-311.

[30] C. M. Beall, G. M. Brittenham, K. P. Strohl, et al., Hemoglobin concentration of highaltitude Tibetans and Bolivian Aymara, Am. J. Phys. Anthropol.106(1998)385-400.

[31] L. G. Moore, F. Armaza, M. Villena, et al., Comparative aspects of high-altitude adaptation in human populations, Adv. Exp. Med. Biol.475(2000) 45-62.

[32] L. G. Moore, D. Young, R. E. McCullough, et al., Tibetan protection from intrauterine growth restriction(IUGR) and reproductive loss at high altitude, Am. J. Hum. Biol.13(2001) 635-644.

西藏林芝、拉萨、安多3个不同海拔区县高血压患者用药情况分析△

张林峰，王增武，陈　祚，王　馨，董　莹，聂静雨，王佳丽，郑聪毅，田　野，邵　澜，朱曼璐

中国医学科学院阜外医院，国家心血管病中心社区防治部　北京 . 102308

通讯作者：王增武，E-mail：wangzengwu@foxmail.com

摘　要　目的　探讨西藏3个区县高血压患者的用药情况。**方法**　2014～2016年在西藏林芝县（海拔3 000 m）、拉萨市区（海拔3 650 m）、安多县（海拔4 700 m）每个区县随机抽取社区居民1 000人进行心血管病患病率调查，对检出的有高血压史的患者的用药情况进行分析。**结果**　3个区县共检出有高血压史的患者490例（林芝县148例、拉萨市190例、安多县152例），2周内经常服用降压药者的比例均＜40.0%，2周内经常服用降压药者的血压控制率均＜50.0%。在高血压患者使用的药物中，藏药和中成药占相当大的比重，占各类药物使用频次的36.84%。拉萨市区有72.55%的患者单用藏药进行降压治疗，该地区2周内经常服用降压药患者的血压控制率仅为15.7%。**结论**　西藏地区高血压患者的药物治疗状况不容乐观，亟需对药物治疗现状进行进一步的深入分析并开展规范化的管理和治疗。

关键词　西藏；高血压；药物治疗

Analysis of the Antihypertensive Drug Usage and Effectiveness in Three Counties with Different Altitudes in Tibet Autonomous Region in China

Zhang Linfeng, Wang Zengwu, Chen Zuo, Wang Xin, Dong Ying, Nie Jingyu, Wang Jiali, Zheng Congyi, Tinan Ye, Shao Lan, Zhu Manlu

Department of Prevention and Community Health, Fuwai Hospital, Chinese Academy of Medical

---

△　本文发表于：中华高血压杂志，2017，25（7）：643-648.

Science, National Center for Cardiovascular Disease, Beijing 102308, China

Abstract **Objective** To explore the usage and effectiveness of the antihypertensive drugs in three counties or districts in Tibet Autonomous Region in China. **Methods** Surveys on the prevalence of major cardiovascular disease were conducted in Linzhi county (altitude 3 000 meters), Chengguan district of Lasa city (altitude 3 650 meters), and Anduo county (altitude 4 700 meters) from 2014 to 2016. One thousand residents were randomly selected from each county/district and the information on cardiovascular disease, related risk factors and drug usage data were collected. The antihypertensive drug usage and effectiveness of the hypertensive patients were analyzed. **Results** A total of 490 hypertensive patients were identified during the surveys, among whom 148 were from Linzhi county, 190 from Chengguan district, and 152 from Anduo county. For the three counties/district, the proportions of the patients taking antihypertensive drugs regularly in the nearest two weeks were all below 40.0% and the control rates of hypertension for these patients were all below 50.0%. The drugs used most frequently were Tibetan and Chinese herbs, which accounted for 36.84% of all the drugs used. In Chengguan district, 72.55% of the patients took only Tibetan herbs and the control rate of hypertension for the patients taking antihypertensive drugs in the nearest two weeks was 15.7%. **Conclusions** The situation is not ideal for the drug therapy of hypertension in Tibet. It is needed to carry out extensive research on the drug therapy and to promote the standardized treatment and management of hypertensive patients in Tibet.

Key words Tibet; hypertension; anti-hypertensive drug

高血压是脑卒中最主要的危险因素，也是冠状动脉性心脏病（冠心病）、心力衰竭及肾病的重要危险因素[1，2]，良好的血压控制可显著减少高血压患者脑卒中、心肌梗死等心脑血管事件的发生，同时可以有效降低死亡风险[3，4]。合理的药物治疗是控制高血压的重要手段。西藏地处我国西南边疆高海拔地区，自然环境特殊，了解当地高血压患者的药物治疗现状对于制定卫生政策、提高当地患者的血压控制水平，改善预后具有重要意义。西藏地区人群中高血压患者的药物治疗现况如何，目前相关研究还较缺乏。本研究将利用公益性行业科研专项“西藏与新疆地区慢性心肺疾病现况调查研究”的资料对这一问题进行初步分析。

1. 对象与方法

1.1 对象

在西藏林芝地区林芝县（海拔 3 000 m）、拉萨市区（海拔 3 650 m）、那曲地区安多县（海拔 4 700 m）3 个区县抽取年龄 > 15 岁常住居民进行调查，在每个区县采用简单随机抽样的方法抽取乡镇（或街道）以及村，再在抽中的村（或居委会）中分性别、年龄采用简单随机抽样的方法抽取年龄 > 15 岁常住居民进行调查，每个区县调查 1 000 人。本文主要对调查中检出的既往有高血压史的患者的用药情况进行分析。

1.2 方法

1.2.1 一般资料收集 调查采用统一编写的与国际标准化方法相一致的调查方案及调查表格。调查于 2014 ~ 2016 年进行。内容包括：一般状况，生活习惯如吸烟、饮酒状况等，个人和家族病史，高血压患者降压药服用情况，并测量血压、身高、体质量、体脂和腰围，以及进行心电图、X 线胸片和心脏超声检查与血脂血糖等血尿标本的测定。各人群的主要调查人员、质控人员以及资料录入人员在调查前均经过统一培训和考核。血压测量采用统一提供的电子血压计（欧姆龙 HBP-1300），统一在上午进行，调查前通知调查对象正常饮水及服药，要求坐位测量 3 次，收缩压和舒张压取 3 次测量的平均值进行分析。

1.2.2 降压药资料收集和分类 患者是否有高血压由调查员当面询问调查对象获得，高血压需既往经过医生诊断。高血压患者服用的降压药为 2 周内正在服用的降压药，用药情况由调查员通过面对面询问的方式获得，对于调查对象不能提供明确信息的，通过药盒、处方、社区医生等进行核实。经常服药是指≥ 5 次 / 周，偶尔服药指 < 5 次 / 周。在进行药物的组合应用分析时，不同种类的化学药物按其所含的活性成分进行归类，如使用固定配比复方制剂，则按照所含的活性成分算 1 种药，藏药和中成药则不区分具体组成分为 1 类。在进行药物的类别分析时，依据《中国高血压防治指南 2010》将化学药根据活性成分分为钙离子通道阻滞剂、血管紧张素转换酶抑制剂、血管紧张素受体阻滞剂、利尿剂、β 受体阻滞剂进行分析 [5]，不在上述 5 类化学降压药中的 α 受体阻滞剂、中枢性降压药等则归为其他降压药，藏药和中成药则合作一类进行分析，不同种类药物的使用情况根据药物使用频次进行统计，如 1 例患者使用 2 种药，则每种药各统计 1 次，如使用固定配比复方制剂，则按照活性成分归类，每种活性成分各统计 1 次，包含中药成分的复方中成药，不计算中药成分，按照其包含的西药活性成分统计分类。

1.2.3 相关指标定义 吸烟是最近 1 个月仍在吸烟者；饮酒是指最近 1 个月每周至少饮酒 1 次者。体重指数（body mass index，BMI）按体重（kg）/ 身高平方（m^2）计算，超重定义为 BMI ≥ 24 且 < 28 kg/m^2，肥胖定义为 BMI ≥ 28 kg/m^2，腹型肥胖定义为腰围≥ 85 cm（男性）、≥ 80 cm（女性）[6]。文化程度中包括肄业者（如初中包括初中未毕业者）。冠心病史、脑卒中史、糖尿病史、慢性心力衰竭史指既往有过医生诊断者，冠心病包括心肌梗死、冠状动脉旁路移植和支架植入 3 种事件中的一种或多种。血压控制达标的判断标准依据《中国高血压防治指南 2010》[5] 及《老年高血压特点与临床诊治流程专家建议》[7]，血压控制达标的标准为：年龄 < 65 岁成人血压 < 140/90 mmHg，患有糖尿病或冠心病者血压 < 130/80 mmHg；年龄≥ 65 岁的患者血压 < 150/90 mmHg，患有糖尿病、冠心病、心力衰竭者血压 < 140/ 90 mmHg。控制率是指调查时检测的血压达到控制标准的人数占总人数的比例。

1.3 资料整理和统计学方法

资料通过平板电脑进行收集并及时上传和核实，所有资料均经逻辑核对后进行分析。分类变量以构成比或率表示，比较采用卡方检验，连续性变量以均数 ± 标准差（$\bar{x}$ ± SD）表示，组间比较采用方差分析。所有统计采用 SAS 9.4 软件进行，以 P < 0.05 为差异有统计学意义。

2. 结果

2.1 研究对象一般情况

林芝县、拉萨市区和安多县一共检出既往有高血压史的患者 490 例，其中林芝县 148 例、拉萨市区 190 例、安多县 152 例。研究对象中藏族的比例均 > 90.0%，最高的是安多县，为 97.4%。3 个区县研究对象的文化程度均以未上学和小学文化程度者居多，均 > 80.0%。研究人群的腹型肥胖率均 > 70.0%，最高的为拉萨市区（81.5%）。3 个区县研究对象的年龄、男性比例、文化程度构成、饮酒率、BMI、收缩压、舒张压、冠心病史、脑卒中史和糖尿病史差异有统计学意义，见表 1。

2.2 研究对象 1 年内和近 2 周的降压药服用与血压达标情况

3 个区县 1 年内经常服用降压药者的比例均 < 50.0%，最低的拉萨市区为 38.4%，2 周内经常服用降压药者的比例均 < 40.0%（表 2）。除安多县未服药组人群的血压控制率 > 50.0% 外，其余各组人群的血压控制率均 < 50.0%，最低者仅为 13.8%。安多县未服药组和经常服药组人群的血压控制率高于另两个区县（$P < 0.01$）。另外从数值上看林芝县 2 周内经常服用降压药者其血压的控制率高于不服用降压药者，而拉萨市区和安多县经常服用降压药者其血压的控制率甚至低于不服用降压药者，但在这 3 个地区，2 周内未服药者、偶尔服药者和经常服药者血压控制率的差异无统计学意义（均 $P > 0.05$）（表 2）。

表 1 研究人群的基本特征

县 / 市	例数	年龄（岁）	男性 [例（%）]	藏族 [例（%）]	小学及以下文化 [例（%）]	吸烟 [例（%）]	饮酒 [例（%）]
林芝县	148	58.4 ± 10.9	68（46.0）	142（96.0）	160（84.2）	26（17.6）	10（6.8）
拉萨市区	190	57.8 ± 10.5	65（34.2）	178（93.7）	125（82.2）	26（13.7）	12（6.3）
安多县	152	53.5 ± 16.7	75（49.3）	148（97.4）	136（91.9）	29（19.1）	2（1.3）
P 值		0.001	0.011	0.251	0.038	0.378	0.047

续表

县 / 市	收缩压（mmHg）	舒张压（mmHg）	BMI（kg/m²）*	腰围（cm）*	超重[例（%）]*	肥胖[例（%）]*
林芝县	155.8 ± 23.2	95.1 ± 13.6	26.2 ± 4.1	88.8 ± 13.0	53（37.9）	45（32.1）
拉萨市区	154.5 ± 21.2	93.8 ± 12.8	27.1 ± 3.9	91.6 ± 10.7	73（38.8）	77（41.0）
安多县	139.5 ± 24.9	88.8 ± 16.6	27.5 ± 4.4	91.3 ± 11.7	46（31.5）	63（43.1）
P 值	< 0.001	< 0.001	0.028	0.075	0.347	0.127

县 / 市	腹型肥胖[例（%）]*	冠心病史[例（%）]	脑卒中史[例（%）]	糖尿病史[例（%）]	心力衰竭史[例（%）]	心血管病家族史[例（%）]
林芝县	108（73.5）	0	0	1（0.7）	1（0.1）	60（40.5）
拉萨市区	154（81.5）	0	8（4.2）	11（5.8）	2（1.1）	92（48.2）
安多县	114（76.0）	3（2.0）	3（2.0）	5（3.3）	0	152（38.2）
P 值	0.196	0.035	0.034	0.038	0.460	0.129

注：计量资料以（$\bar{x}$ ± SD）表示。BMI：体重指数。*3 组 BMI 数据完整的例数分别为 140、188 和 146 例；腰围数据完整的例数分别为 147、189 和 150 例。冠心病：包括心肌梗死、冠状动脉旁路移植和支架植入。心血管病家族史：父母、兄弟姐妹中有高血压、冠心病、脑卒中、糖尿病者。

表 2　研究人群降压药服用和血压控制情况

时间	服药情况	林芝县（n = 148）例数（%）*	血压控制率（%）	拉萨市区（n = 190）例数（%）*	血压控制率（%）	安多县（n = 152）例数（%）*	血压控制率（%）	*P* 值
1 年内	未服	29（19.6）	13.8	41（21.6）	29.3	48（31.6）	58.3	< 0.001
	偶尔	60（40.5）	15.0	76（40.0）	21.1	41（27.0）	31.7	0.132
	经常	59（39.9）	27.1	73（38.4）	15.1	63（41.4）	41.3	0.003
	P 值		0.170		0.195		0.035	
2 周内	未服	41（27.7）	17.1	46（24.2）	26.1	58（38.2）	53.4	< 0.001
	偶尔	60（40.5）	15.0	74（39.0）	21.6	38（25.0）	31.6	0.003
	经常	47（31.8）	27.7	70（36.8）	15.7	56（36.8）	42.9	0.150
	P 值		0.233		0.383		0.105	

* 括号中数据为服药情况构成比。

2.3 研究对象 2 周内服药情况与血压水平、合并症和舒张末期左心室后壁厚度的关系

总研究人群中 2 周内经常服用降压药者的收缩压水平较高，合并糖尿病、冠心病、脑卒中或心力衰竭者的比例也高于其他两组（$P < 0.05$）（表 3）。超声心动图的结果显示，2 周内经常服药者的舒张末期左心室后壁较厚（$P = 0.049$）（表 3）。

表 3 2 周内服药情况与血压水平、合并症和超声心动图舒张末期左心室后壁厚度的关系

县 / 市	服药情况	收缩压（mmHg）	舒张压（mmHg）	合并症*[例（%）]	舒张末期左心室后壁厚度（mm）
林芝县	未服	157.0 ± 24.7	98.5 ± 12.3	0	10.51 ± 1.54
	偶尔	149.6 ± 20.5	93.0 ± 13.7	0	10.00 ± 1.53
	经常	159.9 ± 23.4	94.5 ± 14.1	2（3.33）	10.81 ± 2.22
	P 值	0.067	0.140	0.338	0.092
拉萨市区	未服	150.9 ± 20.7	92.7 ± 13.3	2（4.35）	9.43 ± 1.06
	偶尔	155.6 ± 20.3	94.7 ± 11.4	8（11.43）	9.56 ± 1.06
	经常	155.8 ± 22.5	93.5 ± 13.7	11（14.86）	9.62 ± 1.16
	P 值	0.415	0.691	0.195	0.671
安多县	未服	133.7 ± 23.5	86.2 ± 16.6	4（6.90）	9.19 ± 1.09
	偶尔	140.8 ± 25.6	89.3 ± 16.1	1（1.79）	9.34 ± 1.69
	经常	146.6 ± 24.6	92.3 ± 17.2	6（15.79）	9.42 ± 1.54
	P 值	0.040	0.203	0.034	0.735
合计	未服	145.7 ± 25.0	91.7 ± 15.2	6（4.14）	9.64 ± 1.34
	偶尔	149.2 ± 22.9	92.5 ± 13.8	9（5.20）	9.60 ± 1.45
	经常	155.2 ± 23.7	93.6 ± 14.6	19（11.05）	9.99 ± 1.78
	P 值	0.002	0.517	0.038	0.049

注：计量资料以（$\bar{x}$ ± SD）表示。* 合并糖尿病、冠心病、脑卒中或心力衰竭。

2.4 研究人群降压药服用情况

3 个区县研究人群中 2 周内经常和偶尔服用降压药的患者分别为 173 和 172 例，由于部分患者不能提供其所用药物的信息，本文对能提供详细用药信息的 192 例患者的用药情况进行了分析。结果显示，研究人群使用的降压药物中藏药占有相当的比例，林芝县、拉萨市和安多县单用藏药降压者的比例分别为 40.74%、72.55% 和 36.78%，从 3 个区县合计来看，应用较多的药物组合为单用藏药、单用复方利血平氨苯蝶啶片和单用中成药，所占的

比例分别为47.40%、16.67%和13.02%，其他药物组合所占的比例合计为22.91%（表4）。如以用药频次计算，各类药物的使用情况排在前3位的药物分别为藏药或中成药、利尿剂和其他降压药（α受体阻滞剂、中枢性降压药等），其应用频次占研究人群各类药物总应用频次的比例分别为36.84%、26.87%和26.04%，其余几类药物（钙离子通道阻滞剂、血管紧张素转换酶抑制剂、血管紧张素受体阻滞剂和β受体阻滞剂）的应用频次合计为10.25%。各个区县不同种类药物的使用情况存在差异，林芝县和安多县的藏药或中成药、利尿剂和其他降压药应用较多，而拉萨市区则藏药或中成药及钙离子通道阻滞剂应用较多（表5）。

表4 研究人群中各种药物的组合应用情况[例（%）]

县/市	例数	藏药	氨苯蝶啶复方利血平	中成药	复方利血平氨苯蝶啶+藏药	硝苯地平	氨氯地平	非洛地平	卡托普利
林芝县	54	22（40.74）	17（31.48）	8（14.81）	1（1.85）	0	1（1.85）	0	0
拉萨市区	51	37（72.55）	0	2（3.92）	0	3（5.88）	2（3.92）	3（5.88）	1（1.96）
安多县	87	32（36.78）	15（17.24）	15（17.24）	6（6.90）	3（3.45）	0	0	2（2.30）
合计	192	91（47.40）	32（16.67）	25（13.02）	7（3.65）	6（3.13）	3（1.56）	3（1.56）	3（1.56）

县/市	复方利血平氨苯蝶啶+卡托普利	复方利血平氨苯蝶啶+尼莫地平	藏药+中成药	依那普利	厄贝沙坦	美托洛尔	尼莫地平	吲达帕胺	氨氯地平+复方利血平氨苯蝶啶
林芝县	0	0	0	2（3.70）	0	1（1.85）	0	1（1.85）	1（1.85）
拉萨市区	0	0	0	0	1（1.96）	0	0	0	0
安多县	2（2.30）	2（2.30）	2（2.30）	0	0	0	1（1.15）	0	0
合计	2（1.04）	2（1.04）	2（1.04）	2（1.04）	1（0.52）	1（0.52）	1（0.52）	1（0.52）	1（0.52）

县/市	氨氯地平+厄贝沙坦	氨氯地平+厄贝沙坦氢氯噻嗪	卡托普利+中成药	硝苯地平+中成药	厄贝沙坦+非洛地平	复方利血平氨苯蝶啶+硝苯地平	复方利血平氨苯蝶啶+藏药+中成药	复方利血平氨苯蝶啶+卡托普利+中成药	卡托普利+氢氯噻嗪+硝苯地平
林芝县	0	0	0	0	0	0	0	0	0
拉萨市区	1（1.96）	1（1.96）	0	0	0	0	0	0	0
安多县	0	0	1（1.15）	1（1.15）	1（1.15）	1（1.15）	1（1.15）	1（1.15）	1（1.15）
合计	1（0.52）	1（0.52）	1（0.52）	1（0.52）	1（0.52）	1（0.52）	1（0.52）	1（0.52）	1（0.52）

表 5　研究人群中各类药物的使用情况 [例（%）]

县 / 市	总频次*	藏药或中成药	利尿剂	钙离子通道阻滞剂	血管紧张素转换酶抑制剂	血管紧张素受体阻滞剂	β 受体阻滞剂	其他降压药
林芝县	113	31（27.43）	39（34.51）	2（1.77）	2（1.77）	0	1（0.88）	38（33.63）
拉萨市区	55	40（72.73）	1（1.82）	10（18.18）	1（1.82）	3（5.45）	0	0
安多县	193	62（32.12）	57（29.53）	10（5.18）	7（3.63）	1（0.52）	0	56（29.02）
合计	361	133（36.84）	97（26.87）	22（6.09）	10（2.77）	4（1.11）	1（0.28）	94（26.04）

* 药物合计使用频次。药物以使用频次计算，如 1 例患者同时使用 2 种药，则每种药各计算 1 次，如使用固定复方制剂，则按照活性成分归类，每种活性成分各统计 1 次。其他降压药包括 α 受体阻滞剂、中枢性降压药等。

3. 讨论

大量循证医学的资料证明，要改善高血压患者的长期预后，绝大多数患者需要终身服用降压药物。本文对西藏林芝地区林芝县、拉萨市区、那曲地区安多县部分高血压患者用药情况的分析结果显示，3 个地区的高血压患者 2 周内经常服用降压药物者的比例均 < 40.0%，1 年内经常服用降压药物的患者比例最高的为安多县（41.4%）。从服用的降压药物分析，单用藏药治疗者占有相当大的比重，拉萨市区的患者中有高达 72.55% 的患者单用藏药进行降压治疗。从血压控制的效果来看，3 个地区 2 周内经常服用降压药者的血压控制率均 < 50.0%，拉萨市区 2 周内经常服用降压药的患者血压控制率仅为 15.7%。

黄立等[8] 2016 年对深圳市龙华新区民治街道的 486 例原发性高血压患者抗高血压药使用调查的分析结果显示，使用单药、两种降压药联用、3 种降压药联用及 4 种降压药联用对原发性高血压的控制率分别为 80.42%、90.23%、90.91% 和 89.13%；2015 年，刘建华等[9]对北京市昌平区所辖山区农村高血压患者的调查表明，在接受药物治疗的 213 例患者中，血压控制达标者 153 例，达标率为 71.8%。而在本研究中西藏 3 个区县 2 周内经常服用降压药者的血压控制率均 < 50.0%。同为社区居民，为什么服药者血压的控制效果会有如此大的差距？进一步的分析显示，这可能与选用的降压药有关。目前临床上常用的降压药有 5 大类，即钙离子通道阻滞剂、血管紧张素转换酶抑制剂、血管紧张素受体阻滞剂、β 受体阻滞剂及利尿剂[5]。在深圳市龙华新区民治街道和北京市昌平区所辖山区农村的高血压患者中，上述药物得到了广泛应用[8-9]。然而，本文数据显示林芝、拉萨和那曲的样本人群中上述药物的应用较少，人群应用最多的药物为藏药和中成药，藏药和中成药占各类降压药使用频次的 36.84%，拉萨市区的患者中有 72.55% 的患者单用藏药进行降压治疗。藏药和中成药对于高血压可能有独特的作用[10]，对此还需进行进一步研究。另外，药物的使用方法和

依从性对于血压的控制效果也有重要影响[11]。苗杰等[12]对西藏堆龙德庆县年龄 > 45 岁高血压患者服药依从性的分析表明，患者服药依从性良好的比例仅占 6.52%，依从性差的比例高达 93.47%，其中有 42.93% 的患者起初因高血压住院或高血压症状门诊就诊，规律服药 1 个月左右，待常规降压药服完后，自觉症状消失或不明显而自行停药或改服藏药。由于抗高血压治疗的获益主要来自于降压本身，降压达标是硬道理[11]，因而，在西藏地区加强基层医务人员和高血压患者的教育和培训对于控制血压和改善预后具有重要意义，不仅要提高患者用药的依从性，还需要教育患者在用药的同时，及时监测用药效果，合理规范地使用降压药物。

本文的数据还显示，经常服用降压药的患者其血压控制率与偶尔服药者和未服药者之间差异无统计学意义，这除了与样本量较小、高血压患者服药治疗不规范及依从性较差有关外，也与患者的病情有关。对研究人群心脏超声数据的分析显示未服药者、偶尔服药者和经常服药者的舒张末期左心室后壁厚度分别为 9.64 mm、9.60 mm 和 9.99 mm，经常服药者合并糖尿病、冠心病、脑卒中或心力衰竭的比例也较高，经常服药者的病情较重；未服药的高血压患者病情较轻，而经常服用降压药的患者病情较重或多属服药效果不好的患者。另外，未服药和偶尔服药者的高血压控制率较高还可能与高海拔引起的血压波动和误诊有关。此外，安多县 2 周内未服药组和经常服药组的血压控制率显著高于另两个区县，这可能是由于安多县海拔较高（海拔 4 700 m，接近人类生存极限），患者的血压可能受到高海拔引起的生理反应的影响因而容易造成误诊。关于这些现象，还有待进一步深入研究。

本研究的对象来自于抽样调查随机抽取的样本人群，有较好的代表性。然而，由于每个区县调查抽取的样本人群为 1 000 人，其中既往经医生诊断有高血压的患者只占一小部分，因而样本量较小。同时，由于西藏地区幅员辽阔、人口稀少，分析的 3 个区县主要集中于人口相对稠密和医疗卫生条件较好的地区，缺少西藏边远地区的样本。另一方面，由于本研究为横断面研究，研究中高血压患者的诊断依靠调查对象自报，难免有信息偏倚，而且，对于现象的成因也无法进行深入的探讨。另外，高血压药物的使用情况也主要依据患者提供信息，而不是医生处方和客观记载，难免有遗漏和错误，因而，准确性尚有待进一步提高。

西藏地区高血压患者的药物治疗状况不容乐观，亟需对高血压患者的药物治疗现状进行进一步的深入分析并开展规范化的管理和治疗。

4. 本主题国内外已有的结论

• 深圳市龙华新区民治街道 486 例原发性高血压患者用单药，2、3 及 4 种降压药联用对原发性高血压的控制率分别为 80.42%、90.23%、90.91% 和 89.13%。

• 刘建华等 2015 年对北京市昌平区所辖山区农村高血压患者的调查表明，在 213 例采取药物治疗者中，血压控制达标者 153 例，达标率为 71.8%。

5. 本文特色与见解

• 西藏林芝县、拉萨市区、安多县的高血压患者周 2 内经常服用降压药物者的比例均 < 40.0%，1 年内经常服用降压药物者的比例最高为 41.4%（安多县）。

• 从服用的降压药物分析，单用藏药治疗者占有相当大的比重，拉萨市区的患者中有高达 72.55% 的患者单用藏药进行降压治疗。

• 从血压控制的效果来看，3 个地区 2 周内经常服用降压药者的血压控制率均 < 50.0%，拉萨市区 2 周内经常服用降压药的患者血压控制率仅为 15.7%。

致谢

感谢参与项目的所有专家及所有调查人员。协作组组成单位及主要调查人员：国家心血管病中心、中国医学科学院阜外医院：王增武、张林峰、陈祚、王馨、邵澜、郭敏、田野、赵天明、范国辉、董莹、聂静雨、王佳丽、郑聪毅、贾秀云、朱曼璐、王文、陈伟伟、高润霖；卫生部北京医院：郭岩斐、孙铁英、王玉霞、柴迪、马雅立、仝亚琪；中国人民解放军总医院：陈韵岱、冯斌、朱庆磊、周珊珊、刘杰、王晶、杨丽娜、杨瑛、段鹏； 新疆维吾尔自治区人民医院：李南方、周玲、张德莲、姚晓光、洪静、索菲亚、曹梅；中国疾病预防控制中心：吴静、石文惠、翟屹、何柳。

参考文献

[1] Forouzanfar MH, Liu P, Roth GA, et al. Global burden of hypertension and systolic blood pressure of at least 110 to 115 mmHg, 1990-2015 [J]. JAMA, 2017, 317(2): 165-182.

[2] He J, Gu D, Wu X, et al. Major causes of death among men and women in China [J]. N Engl J Med, 2005, 353(11): 1124-1134.

[3] Liu L, Zhao Y, Liu G, et al. The felodipine event reduction(FEVER) study: a randomized long-term placebo-controlled trial in Chinese hypertensive patients[J]. J Hypertens, 2005, 23(12): 2157-2172.

[4] SPRINT Research Group, Wright JT Jr, Williamson JD, et al. A randomized trial of intensive versus standard blood-pressure control[J]. N Engl J Med, 2015, 373(22): 2103-2116.

[5] 中国高血压防治指南修订委员会. 中国高血压防治指南 2010[J]. 中华高血压杂志，2011, 19(8): 701-743.

[6] 中国肥胖问题工作组. 中国成人超重和肥胖症预防控制指南（节录）[J]. 营养学报，2004, 26(1): 1-4.

[7] 中华医学会老年医学分会，中国医师协会高血压专业委员会. 老年高血压特点与临床诊治流程专家建议

[J]. 中华高血压杂志，2014, 22(7): 620-628.

[8] 黄立，文春颖，郑春英，等. 社区原发性高血压患者抗高血压药使用调查 [J]. 北方药学，2016, 13(8): 176-177.

[9] 刘建华，杜鹃. 北京市边远山区农村高血压患者用药情况现状调查 [J]. 临床药物治疗杂志，2016, 14(3): 40-43.

[10] 次仁达娃，旺堆. 藏医药对高血压病的防治特点 [J]. 西藏科技，2015, (4): 50-63.

[11] 国家卫生计生委合理用药专家委员会，中国医师协会高血压专业委员会. 高血压合理用药指南 [J]. 中国医学前沿杂志电子版，2015, 7(6): 22-64.

[12] 苗杰，王翠侠，张春阳，等. 西藏堆龙德庆县 45 岁以上高血压患者服药依从性分析 [J]. 包头医学院学报，2013, 29(4): 27-31.

新疆地区≥35岁人群代谢综合征患病率情况调查△

董　莹，王　馨，张林峰，陈　祚，聂静雨，王佳丽，郑聪毅，邵　澜，田　野，王增武，周　玲，李南方

中国医学科学院阜外医院，国家心血管病中心社区防治部　北京．102308
通讯作者：王增武，E-mail：wangzengwu@foxmail.com

摘　要　目的　了解新疆地区≥35岁人群代谢综合征（metabolic syndrome，MS）的患病情况和相关危险因素。**方法**　采用多阶段分层随机抽样的方法，于2015年在新疆地区对3 644名35岁及以上常住居民进行调查，包括问卷调查、体格测量和实验室指标的检测。采用美国胆固醇教育计划成人治疗方案第三次报告（NCEP-ATP Ⅲ）诊断亚裔人群修订的版本作为MS的诊断标准，并通过2010年的人口学情况对其进行标化，采用非条件Logistic回归分析其影响因素。**结果**　调查对象的MS患病率为26.40%（标化率为25.46%）。其中男性的患病率为24.66%（标化率为24.49%），女性为28.00%（标化率为26.18%）。在患有MS人群中，同时有中心性肥胖、血压异常和血脂异常三因素者占34.95%。维吾尔族的患病率最高，为41.18%。相对于无高血压家族史者，有高血压家族史人群患MS的风险更高[OR（95%CI）：1.230（1.037～1.459），P=0.017]。**结论**　新疆成年人MS患病率较高，高血压家族史是MS的危险因素。

关键词　代谢综合征；患病率；危险因素；新疆（维吾尔自治区）

Current Status of Metabolic Syndrome among Adults Aged 35 Years and Above in Xinjiang

Dong Ying, Wang Xin, Zhang Linfeng, Chen Zuo, Nie Jingyu, Wang Jiali, Zheng Congyi, Shao Lan, Tian Ye, Wang Zengwu, Zhou Ling, Li Nanfang
Division of Prevention and Community Health, National Center for Cardiovascular Disease, Fuwai Hospital, Pecking Union Medical College & Chinese Academy of Medical Sciences, Beijing

△　本文发表于：中华疾病控制杂志，2017，21（7）：684-687.

102308, China

Abstract Objective To understand the prevalence and influential factors of metabolic syndrome in Xinjiang adults aged 35 years and above. **Methods** Using a multistage stratified random sampling method, investigations including questionnaire, physical examination and blood test, was conducted among inhabitants aged 35 years and above in Xinjiang on 2015. MS was diagnosed according to the US National Cholesterol Education Program Adult Treatment Panel Ⅲ (NCEP ATP Ⅲ) criteria with modification for Asian population. Prevalence of MS was standardized by 2010 general population and non-conditional logistic regression analysis was followed to analyze the risk factor. **Results** The prevalence of MS was 26.40% (aged-standardized prevalence 25.46%), 24.66% (age-adjusted prevalence 24.49%) for males, and 28.00% (age-adjusted prevalence 26.18%) for females. Among participants with MS, 34.95% were with central obesity, high blood pressure, and dyslipidemia. The prevalence of MS was highest in the Uygur (41.18%). People who have family history of hypertension had higher risk of MS than their counterparts [OR (95%CI): 1.230 (1.037 – 1.459), $P = 0.017$]. **Conclusions** The prevalence of MS is higher in Xinjiang adults. Family history of hypertension is one of the risk factors of MS.

Key words Metabolic syndrome; Prevalence; Risk factor; Xinjiang

代谢综合征（metabolic syndrome，MS）是多种代谢危险因素（肥胖、糖代谢异常或糖尿病、高血压和血脂异常）在个体内聚集的状态[1]。大量研究显示，MS与糖尿病的发生和心血管疾病死亡风险升高密切相关[2, 3]。

国外大量研究显示，MS的患病率呈明显上升趋势[4-5]。我国MS的患病率也呈明显的上升趋势。2008年14省≥20岁46 239名研究对象采用2007年中国成人血脂异常防治指南[6]中JCDCG标准得到年龄标化的MS患病率，男性为25.8%，女性为18.0%；而2010年中国非传染性疾病的调查研究中[7]，采用相同的诊断方法，得到MS的患病率分别为男性27.3%，女性27.5%，明显高于2008年的调查结果。虽然国内有许多关于MS的研究[8-10]，但是关于新疆地区资料相对较少，之前的一些研究也往往针对新疆一个地区或一个民族[11, 12]。本研究采取分层随机抽样的方法在新疆地区抽取7个区县，旨在全面了解新疆地区≥35岁人群MS的患病情况，为MS的防治提供参考。

1. 对象与方法

1.1 研究对象

本研究调查对象来自于2014年公益性行业专项“西藏与新疆地区慢性心肺疾病现状调查研究”。采用多阶段分层随机抽样方法，首先在新疆进行城乡分层，在每层内采用成比例抽样（probability proportional to size，PPS）抽取所需数量的区县。然后在被抽中的区 / 县中采用简单随机抽样（simple random sampling，SRS）抽取 2 个街道 / 乡镇。再在被抽中的街道 / 乡镇中采用 SRS 抽取 3 个村 / 居委会。最后在被抽中的村 / 居委会中采用 SRS 随机抽取调查 15 岁及以上个体。一共抽取 7 个地区，每个地区抽取 1 000 名调查对象。并对 35 岁及以上人群采集了血液标本，故本文利用≥ 35 岁人群（完整数据：3 644 例）进行 MS 患病率分析。本研究通过了中国医学科学院阜外医院伦理委员会批准，研究对象均在签署知情同意书后方可进行调查。

1.2 调查方法

本研究为现况调查。调查前由项目组统一发放手册、方案和问卷。每位调查员在培训合格后方能进行调查。调查问卷内容包括①个人基本情况：性别、年龄、婚姻情况、受教育程度、行为习惯（吸烟、饮酒等）；②个人疾病史：如脑卒中、糖尿病、血脂异常等。体格检查：①血压测量：本次血压测量主要采用电子血压计（欧姆龙 HBP-1300），要求调查对象在测量前静坐 5 分钟，并且在测量前 0.5 小时内禁止剧烈活动或饮兴奋性饮料，选择测量右上臂的血压。需连续测量 3 次，每两次间隔 0.5 分钟，将 3 次的均值作为个体的血压值；②身高、体重的测量：体重测量采用体重体脂仪（欧姆龙 V-BODYHBF-371）。实验室标本采集：采集空腹 12 小时血标本，测量空腹血糖（fasting plasma glucose，FPG）、总胆固醇（total cholesterol，TC）、甘油三酯（triglyceride，TG）、高密脂蛋白胆固醇（high-density lipoprotein cholesterol，HDL-C）等生化指标。所有的实验室指标将由统一的实验室进行检测。

1.3 诊断标准

（1）吸烟：一生中吸烟超过 20 包，或每天吸 1 支或以上且连续 1 年及以上。

（2）饮酒：近 1 个月每周至少饮 1 次酒。

（3）糖尿病：FPG ≥ 7.0 mmol/L，或之前确诊为糖尿病并且服用降糖药。

（4）高血压：收缩压（systolic blood pressure，SBP）≥ 140 mmHg 和 / 或舒张压（diastolic blood pressure，DBP）≥ 90 mmHg，或近两周服用降压药。

（5）MS[2，13]：根据美国胆固醇教育计划成人治疗方案第三次报告（NCEP-ATP Ⅲ）（亚裔人群修订版本）：符合下列 3 项及以上者：①中心性肥胖：腰围≥ 90 cm（男性）或≥ 80 cm（女性）；②高 TG 血症：TG ≥ 1.70 mmol/L（150 mg/dl）；③低 HDL-C 血症：HDL-C-C < 1.04 mmol/L（40 mg/dl）（男）或 < 1.30 mmol/L（50 mg/dl）（女）；④ 血压异常：SBP/DBP ≥ 130/85 mmHg；⑤ 血糖异常：FPG ≥ 5.6 mmol/L（100 mg/dl）。在 MS 各指标分析时将高 TG 或低 HDL-C 称为血脂异常。

1.4 统计分析

计量资料使用 $\overline{X} \pm SD$ 表示，两组间均数比较采用 t 检验，多组间比较采用 ANOVA 检验；计数资料用率表示，组间比较采用 χ^2 检验。标化患病率按照 2010 年全国人口普查数据进行标化。影响因素分析采用多因素 Logistic 回归。采用 SAS9.3 进行统计分析，检验水准 $\alpha = 0.05$。

2. 结果

2.1 调查人群的基本特征

本研究中有效样本 3 644 例，年龄为（54.28 ± 13.35）岁，其中男性 1 744 人，占 47.86%。HDL-C 水平、有高血压家族史、吸烟率、饮酒率、已婚比例、汉族比例、文化程度、空腹血糖值和腰围值在男、女之间差异均有统计学意义（均为 $P < 0.05$），见表 1。

表 1　调查对象的基本特征 [n（%）]

特　征	男性（$n = 1\ 744$）	女性（$n = 1\ 900$）	合计（$n = 3\ 644$）	t/χ^2 值	P 值
文化程度					
小学及以下	890（51.03）	1 167（61.42）	2 057（56.45）	42.571	< 0.001
中学	771（44.21）	643（33.84）	1 414（38.80）		
大学及以上	83（4.76）	90（4.74）	173（4.75）		
民族					
汉族	967（55.45）	920（48.42）	1 887（51.78）	37.187	< 0.001
蒙古族	150（8.60）	201（10.58）	351（9.63）		
回族	114（6.54）	150（7.89）	264（7.24）		
维吾尔族	51（2.92）	51（2.68）	102（2.80）		
哈萨克族	142（8.14）	251（13.21）	393（10.78）		
柯尔克孜族	320（18.35）	327（17.21）	647（17.76）		
已婚	1 664（95.41）	1 729（91.00）	3 393（93.11）	27.610	< 0.001
城市居民	570（32.68）	575（30.26）	1 145（31.42）	2.472	0.116
吸烟	1 047（60.03）	121（6.37）	1 168（32.05）	1 202.495	< 0.001
饮酒	279（16.00）	16（0.84）	295（8.10）	280.729	< 0.001

续表

特　征	男性（n＝1 744）	女性（n＝1 900）	合计（n＝3 644）	t/χ^2 值	P 值
年龄（岁）	53.93 ± 13.57	54.57 ± 13.14	54.28 ± 13.35	－1.380	0.168
空腹血糖(mmol/L)	5.49 ± 1.53	5.35 ± 1.37	5.42 ± 1.45	2.920	0.003
HDL-C（mmol/L）	1.30 ± 0.29	1.45 ± 0.29	1.38 ± 0.30	－14.820	＜0.001
腰围（cm）	90.41 ± 0.63	87.24 ± 11.43	88.76 ± 11.17	8.680	＜0.001
高血压	572（32.80）	675（35.53）	1 247（34.22）	3.007	0.083
糖尿病	143（8.20）	150（7.89）	293（8.04）	0.114	0.735
高血压家族史	540（30.96）	677（35.63）	1 217（33.40）	8.909	0.003
血脂异常家族史	124（7.11）	160（8.42）	284（7.79）	2.175	0.140

2.2　不同特征人群 MS 患病率情况

MS 的患病率随年龄的增高而增高（Z = －9.048，P < 0.001），35 岁及以上人群粗患病率为 26.40%，标化患病率为 25.46%；其中男性粗率为 24.66%，标化患病率 24.49%；女性分别为 28.00%、26.18%。男性 55 ~ 64 岁年龄段 MS 患病率最高，而女性的患病率随年龄的增长而升高（Z = －10.192，P < 0.001），见图 1。维吾尔族人群、城市和有高血压家族史者 MS 患病率较高（均为 P < 0.05），见表 2。

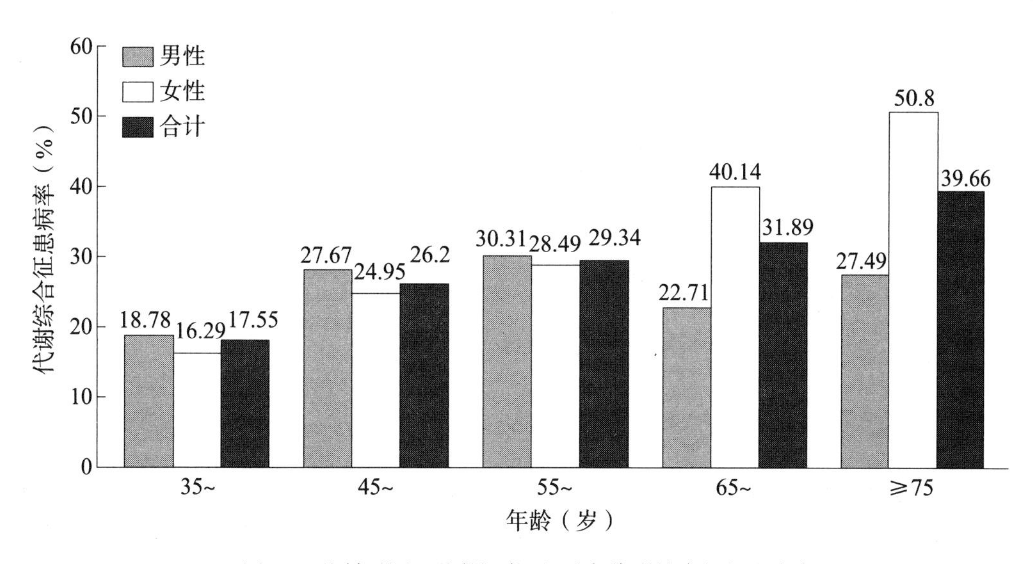

图 1　不同年龄段不同性别调整对象代谢综合征粗患病率

表 2　不同特征人群的代谢综合征患病率

特　　征	患病人数	粗率（%）	标化率（%）	χ^2 值	P 值
性别					
男	430	24.66	24.49	5.233	0.022
女	532	28.00	26.18		
民族					
汉族	592	31.37	29.46	113.224	< 0.001
蒙古族	56	15.95	16.64		
回族	94	35.61	34.79		
维吾尔族	42	41.18	40.14		
哈萨克族	63	16.03	15.97		
柯尔克孜族	115	17.77	17.10		
居住地					
城市	373	32.58	31.30	32.785	< 0.001
农村	589	23.57	22.54		
有无高血压家族史					
无	615	25.34	23.58	4.200	0.040
有	347	28.51	28.90		

2.3　MS 主要指标及其组合比例

在患有 MS 人群中进行了 MS 主要指标的比例计算，发现中心肥胖所占的比例最高，为 94.59%；血压异常和血脂异常分别为 80.35% 和 77.34%；血糖异常为 59.88%。在人群中，发现同时有中心性肥胖、血脂异常和血压异常三种指标的比例最高，为 34.95%；此外，同时有血脂异常、血压异常和血糖异常者的比例最低，为 4.01%。

2.4　MS 的多因素分析

单因素分析有统计学意义的变量进一步以是否患 MS 为因变量（0 = 否；1 = 是）进行多因素 Logistic 回归分析。结果显示，女性、高龄、有高血压家族史者患 MS 的风险较高（均有 $P < 0.05$）。研究也发现与汉族相比，维吾尔族和回族人的患病风险较高（均为 $P < 0.05$），见表 3。

表 3　代谢综合征影响因素的多因素 Logistic 回归分析

特　征	β	sx	OR（95%CI）值	P 值
性别				
男			1.000	
女	0.266	0.098	1.304（1.075 ~ 1.582）	0.007
年龄（岁）				
35 ~			1.000	
45 ~	0.501	0.110	1.651（1.330 ~ 2.049）	< 0.001
55 ~	0.673	0.120	1.961（1.551 ~ 2.480）	< 0.001
65 ~	0.810	0.128	2.248（1.751 ~ 2.888）	< 0.001
≥ 75	1.115	0.141	3.050（2.314 ~ 4.020）	< 0.001
民族				
汉族			1.000	
蒙古族	− 0.667	0.163	0.513（0.373 ~ 0.707）	< 0.001
回族	0.278	0.141	1.321（1.002 ~ 1.742）	< 0.001
维吾尔族	0.524	0.216	1.689（1.106 ~ 2.579）	< 0.001
哈萨克族	− 0.812	0.153	0.444（0.329 ~ 0.599）	< 0.001
柯尔克孜族	− 0.640	0.127	0.527（0.411 ~ 0.676）	< 0.001
高血压家族史				
否			1.000	
是	0.207	0.087	1.230（1.037 ~ 1.459）	0.017

3. 讨论

本研究采用了 NCEP-ATP Ⅲ对新疆地区 MS 的患病情况进行分析，结果显示，新疆地区≥ 35 岁人群 MS 的患病率为 26.40%，标化患病率为 25.46%。多因素分析提示，女性、高龄、有高血压家族史者 MS 的发生风险相对较高，维吾尔族和回族人的患病风险要高于汉族。

由于城镇化、工业化、人口老龄化和人们生活方式的改变，我国 MS 的患病率呈明显上升趋势，有研究[14]对比了 2009 年与 2004 ~ 2005 年 15 个地区的 35 ~ 59 岁 MS 的患病率变化特征，结果发现 MS 标化率从 7.2% 增加到 10.0%。2007 年新疆三地区 3 252 例

20～74 岁成年人 MS 调查（NCEP-ATP Ⅲ标准）显示男性的标化患病率为 22.0%，女性为 24.6%[15]。本次研究无论男性（标化率 24.49%）、女性（标化率 26.18%），均较前增高。因此，新疆地区 MS 的危害同样需要重视。

总体来看，MS 的患病率随年龄的升高而升高[16-17]，此外，年龄、性别分层分析发现，男性 55～64 岁 MS 的患病率达到最高，而女性患病率随年龄呈上升趋势，与之前日本的研究结果相近[18]。对 MS 的各指标分析发现，血脂异常、血压异常和血糖异常在 55～65 岁的年龄段，女性的患病率明显超过男性，可能是因为女性绝经导致各种代谢异常[19-20]。

就民族而言，新疆是一个多民族的聚居地，其地理环境和生活习惯与其他省份大不相同。李春晖[21]的研究显示，无论使用何种诊断标准，维吾尔族人的 MS 患病率均高于其他民族，本次研究也得到了相同的结论。本文中涉及到的 6 个民族，维吾尔族的患病率最高，为 41.18%，经标化后其患病率（40.14%）依然高于其他民族。此外，多因素 Logistic 回归也提示维吾尔族患病风险高。可能与该民族特殊的饮食习惯密切相关，维吾尔族居民日常以碳水化合物为主，冬季畜肉摄入较多，蔬菜水果摄入相对较少，因而维生素 C、β-胡萝卜素、多酚类等对心血管有保护作用的因子也就较少[22]。此外，根据 MS 各指标的单独分析发现，对 MS 影响较大的指标如中心性肥胖、血脂异常和血压异常等，在维吾尔族人群中的患病率均高于其他民族。这在一定程度上解释了其 MS 患病率高的原因。MS 具多种危险因素聚集的特征，其中每一指标都会增加心血管病的发生风险，但多种合并在一起心血管病的发生风险更大[14]。本研究显示，中心性肥胖、血压异常和血糖异常是排名前 3 的指标。就多组分组合来看，中心性肥胖、血脂异常和血压异常的比重最高，占全部 MS 的 34.95%，故建议在新疆地区进行 MS 的防治时应以肥胖、血脂异常和血压异常为主，进行综合干预和管理。

本次研究的优势在于，采用多阶段分层随机抽样的方法选取调查对象，使结果具有较好的代表性。然而，其中也存在一定局限性。由于条件的限制，本研究只针对≥ 35 岁的人群进行了血标本等实验室指标的检查，故只能代表 35 岁及以上人群 MS 患病率的情况。其次，未进行详细的膳食行为调查，不能详细分析膳食行为的影响。此外，本研究为横断面研究，不能得到以上危险因素与 MS 之间的因果关系。

总体上，新疆地区的 MS 患病率处于较高水平，女性、高龄、高血压家族史阳性者为高危人群，中心性肥胖组份贡献最大。应重视该人群，在实际工作中加强肥胖、血脂异常和血压异常的预防和干预，以降低 MS 的发生风险。

致谢

感谢协作组组成单位及主要调查人员：国家心血管病中心、中国医学科学院阜外医院：王增武、张林峰、陈祚、王馨、邵澜、郭敏、田野、赵天明、范国辉、董莹、聂静雨、王佳丽、郑聪毅、贾秀云、朱曼璐、王文、陈伟伟、高润霖；卫生部北京医院：郭岩斐、孙铁英、王玉霞、柴迪、马雅立、仝亚琪；中国人民解放军总医院：陈韵岱、冯斌、朱庆磊、周珊珊、刘杰、王晶、杨丽娜、杨瑛、段鹏；新疆维吾尔自治区人民医院：李南方、周玲、张德莲、姚晓光、洪静、索菲亚、曹梅；中国疾病预防控制中心：吴静、石文惠、翟屹、何柳。

参考文献

[1] Han TS, Lean ME. A clinical perspective of obesity, metabolic syndrome and cardiovascular disease [J]. JRSM Cardiovasc Dis, 2016, 5: 1-13.

[2] Expert Panel on Detection, Evaluation, and Treatment of High Blood Cholesterol in Adults. Executive summary of the third report of the national cholesterol education program(NCEP)expert panel on detection, evaluation, and treatment of high blood cholesterol in adults(Adult Treatment Panel Ⅲ) [J]. JAMA, 2001, 285(19): 2486-2497.

[3] Isomaa B, Almgren P, Tuomi T, et al. Cardiovascular morbidity and mortality associated with the metabolic syndrome [J]. Diabetes Care, 2001, 24(4): 683-689.

[4] Aguilar M, Bhuket T, Torres S, et al. Prevalence of the metabolic syndrome in the United States, 2003-2012 [J]. JAMA, 2015, 313(19): 1973-1974.

[5] Lim S, Shin H, Song JH, et al. Increasing prevalence of metabolic syndrome in Korea: the Korean national health and nutrition examination survey for 1998-2007 [J]. Diabetes Care, 2011, 34(6): 1323-1328.

[6] Hou X, Lu J, Weng J, et al. Impact of waist circumference and body mass index on risk of cardiometabolic disorder and cardiovascular disease in Chinese adults: a national diabetes and metabolic disorders survey [J]. PLoS One, 2013, 8(3): e57319.

[7] Lu J, Wang L, Li M, et al. Metabolic syndrome among adults in China-the 2010 China noncommunicable disease surveillance [J]. J Clin Endocrinol Metab, 2017, 102(2): 507-515.

[8] 丁贤彬，毛德强，沈卓之，等．重庆市成年居民代谢综合征患病率及影响因素 [J]．公共卫生与预防医学，2016, 27(4): 54-58.

[9] 邵永强，樊丽辉，李江峰，等．温州市居民代谢综合征患病率及影响因素调查 [J]．中国慢性病预防与控制，2016, 24(6): 419-422.

[10] 赵天明，王增武，张林峰，等．北方农村 35 岁及以上人群代谢综合征患病情况调查 [J]．中华疾病控制杂志，2015, 19(5): 439-442.

[11] 李春晖，郭淑霞，马儒林，等．2010 年新疆喀什地区维吾尔族人群代谢综合征流行现状 [J]．中华预防医学杂志，2012, 46(5): 419-423.

[12] 张丽，李玉芳，桑晓红，等．4 种代谢综合征诊断标准在农村维吾尔族围绝经期妇女中的应用比较 [J].

新疆医科大学学报，2016, 39(8): 940-943.

[13] Grundy SM, Cleeman JI, Daniels SR, et al. Diagnosis and management of the metabolic syndrome: an American heart association/national heart, lung, and blood institute scientific statement: executive summary[J]. Crit Pathw Cardiol, 2005, 4(4): 198-203.

[14] 王增武，王馨，李贤，等. 中国 35 ~ 59 岁人群代谢综合征患病率及其变化 [J]. 中华流行病学杂志，2009, 30(6): 596-600.

[15] 赵力敏，田晓琴，赵凤丛. 新疆三地区成人代谢综合征患病率调查 [J]. 新疆医学，2010, 40(5): 4-8.

[16] Lee WY, Park JS, Noh SY, et al. Prevalence of the metabolic syndrome among 40, 698 Korean metropolitan subjects[J]. Diabetes Res Clin Pract, 2004, 65(2): 143-149.

[17] Gu D, Reynolds K, Wu X, et al. Prevalence of the metabolic syndrome and overweight among adults in China [J]. Lancet, 2005, 365(9468): 1398-1405.

[18] Kuzuya M, Ando F, Iguchi A, et al. Age-specific change of prevalence of metabolic syndrome: longitudinal observation of large Japanese cohort [J]. Atherosclerosis, 2007, 191(2): 305-312.

[19] Carr MC. The emergence of the metabolic syndrome with menopause [J]. J Clin Endocrinol Metab, 2003, 88(6): 2404-2411.

[20] Eshtiaghi R, Esteghamati A, Nakhjavani M. Menopause is an independent predictor of metabolic syndrome in Iranian women [J]. Maturitas, 2010, 65(3): 262-266.

[21] 李春晖. 新疆地区代谢综合征的研究进展 [J]. 医学综述，2012, 18(10): 1537-1538.

[22] 杨天，马依彤，杨毅宁，等. 新疆地区汉族、维吾尔族成年人群代谢综合征流行病学调查 [J]. 新疆医科大学学报，2011, 34(2): 129-132.

新疆、西藏地区居民肥胖类型与10年冠心病发病风险关系的研究△

郑聪毅，王增武，陈 祚，张林峰，王 馨，董 莹，聂静雨，王佳丽，邵 澜，田 野

中国医学科学院阜外医院，国家心血管病中心社区防治部 北京 . 102308

通讯作者：王增武，E-mail: wangzengwu@foxmail.com

摘 要 目的 探讨我国新疆、西藏地区居民肥胖类型及与10年冠心病发病风险关系。**方法** 采用多阶段分层随机抽样的方法，共抽取新疆、西藏两地≥35岁研究对象7 631人，其中5 802人纳入本研究分析。**结果** 研究对象的普通肥胖、腹型肥胖、内脏肥胖和混合型肥胖患病率分别为0.53%、12.62%、10.08%和42.35%。其中混合肥胖中同时满足3种肥胖类型诊断标准的研究对象占58.65%（1 441/2 457）。男、女性10年冠心病患病风险分别为（3.05 ± 4.14）%和（1.42 ± 2.37）%（男性高于女性，$P < 0.000\ 1$）。混合型肥胖研究对象高等级冠心病发病风险所占比例为30.16%，显著高于普通肥胖（19.35%）、腹型肥胖（28.01%）和内脏肥胖（18.46%）。多因素分析校正混杂因素后显示，混合型肥胖人群10年冠心病发病风险高于其他肥胖类型（OR = 2.889，95%CI：2.525 ~ 3.305），其中BMI和腰围两项指标均异常的研究对象10年冠心病风险更高（OR = 3.168，95%CI：2.730 ~ 3.677）。**结论** 肥胖问题在新疆、西藏地区较严重，男性、混合型肥胖（特别是BMI与腰围均异常）人群10年冠心病发病风险高。

关键词 肥胖类型；混合型肥胖；10年冠心病发病风险；西藏；新疆

Association between the Types of Obesity and the 10-year Coronary Heart Disease Risk in Tibet Autonomous Region and Xinjiang Uygur Autonomous Region

Zheng Congyi, Wang Zengwu, Chen Zuo. Zhang Linfeng, Wang Xin, Dong Ying, Nie Jingyu,

△ 本文发表于：中华流行病学杂志，2017，38（6）：721-726.

Wang juali, Shao Lan, Tian Ye, for the Group of, Study on Prevalence of Chronic Cardiopulmonary Disease in Tibet and Xinjiang Area
Division of Prevention and Community Health, National Center for Cardiovascular Diseases; Fuwai Hospital, PUMC and CAMS, Beijing 102308, China
Corresponding author: Wang Zengwu, Email: wangzengwu@foxmail. com

Abstract **Objective** To investigate the association between types of obesity and the 10-year-coronary heart disease risk in Tibet and Xinjiang of China. **Methods** Using the multi-stage random sampling method, 7 631 participants aged 35 or older were examined under the International Standardized Examination process but with only 5 802 were eligible for analysis in the 2015-2016 season. **Results** The prevalence rates of general obesity, central obesity, visceral obesity and compound obesity were 0.53%, 12.62%, 10.08% and 42.35%, respectively. Out of all the compound obesity cases, 58.65% (1 441/2 457) of them appeared as having all types of obesity in our study. Risk related to the 10-year coronary heart disease was higher in men than in women [(3.05 ± 4.14)% vs (1.42 ± 2.37)%, $P < 0.000$]. Compound obesity (30.16%) showed the highest proportion on the risk of 10-year coronary heart disease than central obesity (28.01%), visceral obesity (18.46%), or general obesity (19.35%). After adjustment for confounding factors, results from the multivariate analysis showed the risk in compound obesity was higher than central obesity, visceral obesity or general obesity and was associated with the highest risk on the 10-year coronary heart disease (OR = 2.889, 95%CI: 2.525 – 3.305). People with anomalous BMI and WC seemed to have had the higher risk(OR = 3.168, 95%CI: 2.730 – 3.677). **Conclusions** Obesity is popular in the residents of Tibet and Xinjiang areas of China. Men and people with compound obesity (especially both BMI and WCwere abnormal) may carry greater risk on the 10-year coronary heart disease.

Key words Obesity type; Compound obesity; 10-year coronary heart disease risk; Tibet; Xinjiang

冠心病是全球，特别是发达国家，危害人类健康的主要疾病，在发展中国家冠心病患病率与国家发展指数成正[1]。我国 2002 ~ 2014 年冠心病死亡率呈上升趋势，2014 年中国冠心病死亡率城市为 107.5/10 万，农村为 105.37/10 万[2]。肥胖是包括冠心病在内的心血管疾病、糖尿病和恶性肿瘤的重要危险因素，严重增加全球疾病负担[3-4]。1991 ~ 2011 年，我国成年人群超重、肥胖患病率呈持续的上升趋势，2011 年超重或肥胖达到 44.0%，2009 年中心性肥胖患病率达到 45.3%[5]。我国中老年人超过半数为超重或肥胖[6]，新疆地区肥胖人群比例显著高于全国水平[7]，西藏地区居民肥胖情况少有报道。国内外研究显示，肥胖是诱发冠心病的高危因素，可增加冠心病患病风险 0.5 ~ 1.0 倍，而且约 23% 的冠心病由肥胖引起[8-9]，但关于不同肥胖类型对冠心病发病风险的影响尚不清楚。因此，本研究利用公益性行业科研专项“西藏与新疆地区慢性心肺疾病现状调查研究”的相关数据，分析新疆、西藏两地 35 岁及以上居民肥胖类型，并探讨肥胖类型与 10 年冠心病发病风险的关系，为制定西部地区包括冠心病在内的心血管疾病防治策略提供科学依据。

1. 对象和方法

1.1 研究对象

本研究是公益性行业科研专项“西藏与新疆地区慢性心肺疾病现状调查研究”的一部分。该研究在我国新疆、西藏两地区采用分层 4 阶段随机抽样方法抽取调查对象。首先分别在西藏自治区和新疆维吾尔自治区内按城乡分为两层，在每层内采用与容量大小成比例的概率（probability proportional to size，PPS）抽取所需数量的区 / 县。然后在每个被抽中的区 / 县中采用简单随机抽样（simple random sampling，SRS）方法抽取两个街道 / 乡镇。再在每个被抽中的街道 / 乡镇中采用 SRS 法抽取 3 个居委会 / 村委会。最后在被抽中的居委会 / 村委会中分性别、年龄采用 SRS 方法随机抽取调查个体。该项目在西藏抽取 6 个区 / 县，在新疆抽取 7 个区 / 县，每个区 / 县样本量为 15 岁及以上对象 1 000 人，其中西藏与新疆地区 35 岁及以上人群分别占 49.6% 和 44.9%。本研究实际入选 35 岁及以上调查对象 7 631 人，其中 5 802 人纳入分析（其中排除确诊或存在既往史的冠心病患者）。

1.2 问卷调查和体格检查

采用统一的方案、手册及问卷，问卷内容包括调查对象个人基本情况、调查对象个人健康状况、主要慢性病的病史资料。体格检查以调查居委会 / 村委会为单位集中进行，各单位测量工具及方法一致，内容包括身高、体重、体脂、腰围、血压、肺功能、血氧饱和度等项目。

1.3 实验室检测

在医学体检的同时，采集调查对象的空腹血液样品，分别测定空腹血糖（FPG），血脂：TG、HDL-C 和 TC，血肌酐，血钾等。所有的血液样品离心、分离血清，－70℃低温冰箱保存，在本区 / 县完成调查后及早运送到项目办公室，到选定的中心实验室统一进行检测。

1.4 质量控制

现场调查前，本课题组成员对各地区调查骨干和人员进行严格培训和考核，并进行为期 1 周的现场督导；为确保各环节的质量，现场调查设有固定的质量控制人员；为确保调查数据和体格检查数据的质量，本研究统一采用现场 Pad 录入并随时上传调查数据，及时数据核查和反馈，为再次询问调查对象、核实信息、调查项目补漏等工作提供可行和便利条件。

1.5 指标定义和标准

（1）肥胖：普通肥胖：根据《中国成人超重和肥胖症预防与控制指南》肥胖切点，BMI ≥ 28 kg/m^2 为肥胖 [10-11]；腹型肥胖：参考《中国成人血脂异常防治指南（2016 年修订版）》，男性腰围≥ 90 cm，女性≥ 85 cm[12]；内脏肥胖：参考日本人群标准，内脏脂肪面积（VFA）≥ 100 或内脏脂肪指数（VFI）≥ 10 为内脏肥胖 [13]。本研究按照不同的肥胖特征将调查对象分为 5 类：①普通肥胖：腰围和内脏脂肪指数正常，但 BMI ≥ 28 kg/m^2；②腹型肥胖：BMI 和内脏脂肪指数正常，但腰围≥ 90 cm（男）/85 cm（女）；③内脏肥胖：BMI 和腰围正常，但 VFA ≥ 100 或 VFI ≥ 10；④混合型肥胖：同时符合以上 2 种或 3 种类型肥胖标准；⑤非肥胖：以上三种肥胖类型标准均不满足。

（2）冠心病发病风险预测模型：本研究中估计 10 年冠心病发病风险的方法为 2004 年发表的中国多省队列研究（Chinese Multi-provincial Cohort Study，CMCS）中 Framingham 校正均值和系数后的预测模型 [14]。不同性别研究对象分别按照 CMCS 中提供的不同参数计算 10 年冠心病发病概率，公式中变量包括：年龄均值、血压水平、TC、HDL-C、是 / 否吸烟和是 / 否糖尿病 6 项指标评估。模型中：①血压水平等级分为理想血压（ < 120/80 mmHg）、正常血压（ < 130/85 mmHg）、正常高值（130 ~ 139/85 ~ 89 mmHg）、Ⅰ级高血压（140 ~ 159/90 ~ 99 mmHg）和Ⅱ ~ Ⅳ级高血压（≥ 160/100 mmHg）共 5 个等级，如果 SBP 和 DBP 分别在不同的血压等级则取最高等级；② TC 分为 < 160、160 ~ 199、200 ~ 239、240 ~ 279 和≥ 280 mg/L 5 个水平；③ HDL-C 分为 < 35、35 ~ 44、45 ~ 49、50 ~ 59 和≥ 60 mg/L 5 个水平；④吸烟者定义为一生中至少吸过 20 且最近 1 个月仍在吸烟；⑤糖尿病定义为既往确诊或实验室检查 FPG ≥ 7.0 mmol/L。

自然人群中的 10 年冠心病风险大多集中在 < 5%，故本研究采用四分位法将 10 年冠心病发病风险由低至高分为 4 等级。

1.6 统计学分析

采用 SAS9.3 软件进行统计分析。计量资料采用均数 ± 标准差（$\bar{x}$ ± SD）进行描述，组间均数比较用两独立样本 t 检验或者 one-way ANOVA 方差分析（SNK 进行两两比较）；组间率的比较用 χ^2 检验；独立样本等级资料比较采用 Kruskal-Wallis 秩和检验。多因素分析采用多元 Logistic 回归分析，本研究采用有序多分类响应变量 Logistic 回归。以双侧检验 $P < 0.05$ 为差异有统计学意义。

2. 结果

2.1 一般情况

本研究实际纳入分析对象 5 802 人，其中男性 2 554 人（44.02%），平均年龄（53.16 ±

12.63）岁，汉族占 36.32%（2 107/5 802）。男性受教育程度、吸烟率、饮酒率、DBP 和血糖水平均高于女性，而居住地高海拔比例和高密度脂蛋白胆固醇水平低于女性（$P < 0.000\ 1$）。其他特征不同性别比较差异无统计学意义（表 1）。

表 1　研究对象基本特征

特　征	男性（$n = 2\ 554$）	女性（$n = 3\ 248$）	合计（$n = 5\ 802$）	P 值
年龄（岁，$\bar{x} \pm SD$）	53.40 ± 13.02	52.98 ± 12.32	53.16 ± 12.63	0.209 5
汉族	1 093（42.80）	1 014（31.22）	2 107（36.32）	< 0.000 1
农村人口	1 925（75.3）	2 461（75.77）	4 386（75.59）	0.726 2
文化程度（初中及以上）	1 068（41.82）	983（30.26）	2 051（35.35）	< 0.000 1
居住地海拔（m）				
< 1 000	1 295（50.70）	1 411（43.44）	2 706（46.64）	< 0.000 1
1 000 ~ 3 500	883（34.57）	1 078（33.19）	1 961（33.80）	
≥ 3 500	376（14.72）	759（23.37）	1 135（19.56）	
吸烟	1 110（43.46）	120（3.69）	1 230（21.20）	< 0.000 1
饮酒	1 134（44.40）	469（14.44）	1 603（27.63）	< 0.000 1
血压（mmHg，$\bar{x} \pm SD$）				
SBP	131.10 ± 19.91	131.00 ± 22.17	131.03 ± 21.21	0.801 7
DBP	79.89 ± 12.12	77.32 ± 12.12	78.45 ± 12.19	< 0.000 1
血脂（mg/dl，$\bar{x} \pm SD$）				
TC	179.00 ± 35.37	181.30 ± 37.23	180.26 ± 36.44	0.015 7
HDL-C	51.37 ± 11.76	57.66 ± 11.97	54.90 ± 12.28	< 0.000 1
LDL-C	106.00 ± 29.34	105.50 ± 30.42	105.68 ± 29.95	0.520 0
血糖（mmol/L，$\bar{x} \pm SD$）	5.38 ± 1.69	5.11 ± 1.39	5.23 ± 1.54	< 0.000 1

注：P 值为不同性别间基本特征 t 检验或 χ^2 检验比较结果。饮酒定义为最近 1 个月每周至少饮酒 1 次；SBP：收缩压，DBP：舒张压；TC：总胆固醇，HDL-C：高密度脂蛋白胆固醇，LDL-C：低密度脂蛋白胆固醇。

2.2　不同肥胖类型人群危险因素情况

5 802 名研究对象 BMI 肥胖率为 26.96%（1 564/5 802），中心性肥胖患病率为 53.96%（3 131/5 802）。5 种不同肥胖类型分布情况：非肥胖 1 997 人（34.42%）、普通肥胖 31 人（0.53%）、腹型肥胖 732 人（12.62%）、内脏肥胖 585 人（10.08%）和混合肥胖 2 457

人（42.35%）；其中混合肥胖中同时符合3种肥胖诊断标准的研究对象占58.65%（1 441/2 457），BMI和腰围均异常的研究对象占60.03%（1 475/2 457）。非肥胖者，高血压、TC和糖尿病患病率显著低于肥胖组；混合型肥胖者，高血压和低高密度脂蛋白胆固醇所占比例较大；腹型肥胖者，高胆固醇所占比例较大（表2）。

表2　不同肥胖类型研究对象相关危险因素水平

危险因素	非肥胖（n = 1 997）	普通肥胖（n = 31）	腹型肥胖（n = 732）	内脏肥胖（n = 585）	混合肥胖（n = 2 457）	P 值
年龄（岁，$\bar{x}$ ± SD）	51.10 ± 12.45	51.26 ± 13 33	51.01 ± 11.77	56.67 ± 13.69	54.65 ± 12.39	< 0.000 1[a]
性别						< 0.000 1
男	701（35.10）	14（45.16）	73（9.97）	497（84.96）	1 269（51.65）	
女	1 296（64.90）	17（54.84）	659（90.03）	88（15.04）	1 188（48.35）	
血压水平						< 0.000 1
理想血压	938（46.97）	5（16.13）	267（36.48）	171（29.23）	439（17.87）	
正常血压	384（19.23）	5（16.13）	148（20.22）	125（21.37）	443（18.03）	
正常高值	234（11.72）	12（38.71）	105（14.34）	86（14.70）	391（15.91）	
Ⅰ级高血压	225（11.27）	5（16.13）	125（17.08）	98（16.75）	554（22.55）	
Ⅱ～Ⅳ级高血压	216（10.82）	4（12.90）	87（11.89）	105（17.95）	630（25.64）	
TC（mg/dl）						< 0.000 1
< 160	733（36.71）	6（19.35）	225（30.74）	156（26.67）	574（23.36）	
160～	826（43.16）	14（45.16）	299（40.85）	265（45.30）	1 075（43.75）	
200～	330（16.52）	7（22.58）	160（21.86）	131（22.39）	627（25.52）	
240～	51（2.55）	4（12.90）	43（5.87）	28（4.79）	151（6.15）	
≥ 280	21（1.05）	0（0.00）	5（0.68）	5（0.85）	30（1.22）	
HDL-C（mg/dl）						< 0.000 1
< 35	33（1.65）	1（3.23）	9（1.23）	19（3.25）	74（3.01）	
35～	246（12.32）	3（9.68）	97（13.25）	113（19.32）	575（23.40）	
45～	265（13.27）	3（9.68）	113（15.44）	103（17.61）	461（18.76）	
50～	601（30.10）	14（45.16）	248（33.88）	200（34.19）	768（31.26）	

续表

危险因素	非肥胖（n＝1 997）	普通肥胖（n＝31）	腹型肥胖（n＝732）	内脏肥胖（n＝585）	混合肥胖（n＝2 457）	P值
≥ 60	852（42.66）	10（32.26）	265（36.20）	150（25.64）	579（23.57）	
吸烟	420（21.03）	4（12.90）	46（6.28）	212（36.24）	548（22.30）	< 0.000 1
糖尿病	58（2.90）	1（3.23）	39（5.33）	36（6.15）	250（10.18）	< 0.000 1

注：[a]SNK 两两比较结果显示内脏肥胖的研究对象平均年龄显著高于其他组；TC：总胆固醇，HDL-C：高密度脂蛋白胆固醇；P值为 5 种肥胖类型间各危险因素的方差分析（年龄）、秩和检验（血压水平、TC 和 HDL-C 水平）和χ^2检验（性别、是/否吸烟和是/否糖尿病）比较结果；括号外数据为例数，括号内数据为构成比（%）。

2.3 肥胖类型与 10 年冠心病发病风险关系

本研究男性 10 年冠心病患病风险 [（3.05 ± 4.14）%] 高于女性 [（1.42 ± 2.37）%]（P < 0.000 1）。非肥胖研究人群符合最低水平冠心病发病风险比例者为 35.23%，普通肥胖、腹型肥胖、内脏肥胖和混合型肥胖研究对象符合最高水平冠心病发病风险比例分别为 19.35%、28.01%、18.46% 和 30.16%（表 3）。

表 3　不同肥胖类型研究对象 10 年冠心病发病风险水平比较

肥胖类型	Q1	Q2	Q3	Q4	P值
男性/（$P_{10\text{-CHD}}$）	0.10% ~ 0.68%	0.68% ~ 1.50%	1.50% ~ 3.71%	3.71% ~ 50.44%	
非肥胖	251（35.81）	175（24.96）	136（19.40）	139（19.83）	< 0.000 1
普通肥胖	6（42.86）	2（14.29）	3（21.43）	3（21.43）	
腹型肥胖	28（38.36）	19（26.03）	13（17.81）	13（17.81）	
内脏肥胖	109（21.93）	115（23.14）	132（26.56）	141（28.37）	
混合肥胖	253（19.94）	316（24.90）	361（28.45）	339（26.71）	
女性/（$P_{10\text{-CHD}}$）	0.13% ~ 0.25%	0.25% ~ 0.50%	0.50% ~ 1.45%	1.45% ~ 39.63%	
非肥胖	463（35.73）	350（27.01）	276（21.30）	207（15.97）	< 0.000 1
普通肥胖	5（29.41）	3（17.65）	6（35.29）	3（17.65）	
腹型肥胖	178（27.01）	192（29.14）	161（24.43）	128（19.42）	
内脏肥胖	11（12.50）	13（14.77）	23（26.14）	41（46.59）	
混合肥胖	154（12.96）	250（21.04）	354（29.80）	430（36.20）	
合计/（$P_{10\text{-CHD}}$）	0.10% ~ 0.56%	0.56% ~ 0.93%	0.93% ~ 2.89%	2.89% ~ 50.44%	

续表

肥胖类型	Q1	Q2	Q3	Q4	P值
非肥胖	611（30.60）	548（27.44）	464（23.23）	374（18.73）	<0.000 1
普通肥胖	9（29.03）	7（22.58）	9（29.03）	6（19.35）	
腹型肥胖	115（15.71）	210（28.69）	202（27.60）	205（28.01）	
内脏肥胖	199（34.02）	133（22.74）	145（24.79）	108（18.46）	
混合肥胖	531（21.61）	538（21.90）	647（26.33）	741（30.16）	

注：括号外数据为例数，括号内数据为构成比（%）；Q1～Q4为10年CHD发病风险的四分位区间，Q1表示各层10年CHD发病风险最低的25%区间，Q4表示10年CHD发病风险最高的25%区间；$P_{10\text{-}CHD}$为10年冠心病发病风险；*P*值为5种肥胖类型间不同等级10年冠心病发病风险水平的秩和检验比较结果。

将10年冠心病发病风险四分位进行Logistic多因素分析。模型1中调整年龄、性别和民族3个混杂因素，结果显示，与非肥胖人群相比，腹型肥胖（OR = 1.562，95%CI：1.306～1.868）、内脏肥胖（OR = 1.651，95%CI：1.330～2.051）、混合型肥胖（OR = 2.875，95%CI：2.514～3.288）可显著增加冠心病患病风险；模型2中调整了年龄、性别、民族、饮酒、居住地海拔、受教育程度、农村/城镇户口、冠心病家族史8个10年冠心病发病风险预测模型之外的混杂因素，分析结果表明，混合型肥胖人群10年冠心病发病风险高于其他肥胖类型（OR = 2.889，95%CI：2.525～3.305）。BMI和腰围两项指标均异常的研究对象10年冠心病风险更大（OR = 3.168，95%CI：2.730～3.677），见表4。

表4　不同肥胖类型多因素调整的10年CHD发病风险水平（OR值95%CI）

肥胖类型	男性（*n* = 2 554）	女性（*n* = 3 248）	合计（*n* = 5 802）
模型1			
非肥胖	1 000	1 000	1.000
普通肥胖	2.129（0.691～6.562）	0.903（0.340～2.402）	1.527（0.684～3.411）
腹型肥胖	1.256（0.755～2.090）	1.628（1.345～1.970）	1.562（1.306～1.868）
内脏肥胖	1.563（1.222～1.999）	1.355（0.832～2.206）	1.651（1.330～2.051）
混合肥胖	2.694（2.208～3.286）	2.651（2.242～3.136）	2.875（2.514～3.288）
模型1			
非肥胖	1 000	1 000	1.000
普通肥胖	2.139（0.694～6.597）	0.899（0.337～2.394）	1.527（0.684～3.409）

续表

肥胖类型	男性（n = 2 554）	女性（n = 3 248）	合计（n = 5 802）
腹型肥胖	1.259（0.756 ~ 2.095）	1.631（1.348 ~ 1.974）	1.575（1.317 ~ 1.885）
内脏肥胖	1.561（1.220 ~ 1.997）	1.346（0.826 ~ 2.193）	1.611（1.297 ~ 2.002）
混合肥胖			
BMI + WC 异常 [a]/ 是	3.133（2.488 ~ 3.945）	2.895（2.415 ~ 3.472）	3.144（2.710 ~ 3.647）
BMI + WC 异常 [a]/ 否	2.323（1.848 ~ 2.919）	2.024（1.551 ~ 2.642）	2.435（2.037 ~ 2.912）
模型 2			
非肥胖	1 000	1 000	1.000
普通肥胖	2.406（0.764 ~ 7.574）	0.903（0.399 ~ 1.592）	1.555（0.695 ~ 3.483）
腹型肥胖	1.368（0.820 ~ 2.281）	1.649（1.362 ~ 1.996）	1.573（1.315 ~ 1.882）
内脏肥胖	1.598（1.248 ~ 2.047）	1.383（0.848 ~ 2.254）	1.650（1.329 ~ 2.050）
混合肥胖	2.731（2.233 ~ 3.340）	2.672（2.259 ~ 3.162）	2.889（2.525 ~ 3.305）
模型 2			
非肥胖	1 000	1 000	1.000
普通肥胖	2.430（0.771 ~ 7.662）	0.898（0.337 ~ 2.394）	1.555（0.695 ~ 3.482）
腹型肥胖	1.375（0.824 ~ 2.294）	1.652（1.365 ~ 2.001）	1.588（1.327 ~ 1.900）
内脏肥胖	1.596（1.246 ~ 2.045）	1.374（0.842 ~ 2.241）	1.608（1.294 ~ 1.999）
混合肥胖			
BMI + WC 异常 [a]/ 是	3.260（2.581 ~ 4.116）	2.927（2.440 ~ 3.512）	3.168（2.730 ~ 3.677）
BMI + WC 异常 [a]/ 否	2.298（1.825 ~ 2.895）	2.025（1.551 ~ 2.644）	2.435（2.036 ~ 2.912）

注：非肥胖为对照组。模型 1 调整年龄、性别和民族；模型 2 调整模型 1 + 饮酒、居住地海拔、受教育程度、农村 / 城镇户口、冠心病家族史。[a]BMI + WC 异常：BMI ≥ 28 kg/m^2，同时腰围≥ 90 cm(男)/85 cm(女)。

3. 讨论

冠心病是全球特别是发达国家危害人类健康的主要疾病，在发展中国家冠心病患病率与国家发展指数呈正比 [1]。目前，国内缺乏西藏新疆地区关于 10 年冠心病发病风险预测以及其影响因素相关具有代表性抽样调查的研究数据。本研究中，男、女性 10 年冠心病患病风险分别为（3.05 ± 4.14）% 和（1.42 ± 2.37）%，显著高于 CMCS 队列中男女两性（1.5% 和 0.6%）[11]。5 802 名研究对象 BMI 肥胖率为 26.96%，中心性肥胖患病率为 53.96% 高于全国中年人水平[5]，究其原因可能是因为新疆、西藏两地主要以牛羊肉为主、较少摄入蔬菜水果，高脂肪、高热量、高蛋白的独特饮食方式以及独特的自然环境、文化生活方式等，很可能导致肥胖、血脂紊乱等心血管病危险因素聚集，大大提高其肥胖率[15]。

5 种肥胖类型中，混合型肥胖患病率最高 64.31%，且混合肥胖中同时符合 3 种肥胖诊断标准的研究对象占 58.65%。BMI 和腰围均异常的研究对象占混合肥胖的 60.03%。多因素分析结果表明，混合型肥胖同其他肥胖类型相比 10 年冠心病发病风险更大。与本研究结果类似，有文献报道混合型肥胖与单一类型（普通肥胖、腹型肥胖）相比，更大地增加心血管病危险因素聚集风险（OR = 5.09，95%CI：4.38 ~ 5.90）[16]。其原因可能是混合型肥胖基于综合判断，弥补了单独采用 BMI 和腰围判断的缺点。BMI 忽略了体内瘦组织和脂肪所占的比例[17]，因此对肌肉很发达的运动员或水肿患者，BMI 可能过高估计其肥胖程度；老年人的肌肉与其脂肪组织相比，肌肉组织减少较多，体重指数可能过低估计其肥胖程度。而腰围忽略了身高的混杂，无法区分皮下和内脏脂肪[18]。另外，本研究发现既满足 BMI 又满足腰围肥胖标准的人群，10 年冠心病发病风险最高（OR = 3.168，95%CI：2.730 ~ 3.677）。与既往研究结果相似，使用 BMI 和腰围或可以更好地估计与多种慢性病的关联[11]，提示今后腰围和 BMI 均异常的人群应为心血管疾病预防和控制的重点干预对象。

本研究结果显示在单一肥胖类型的研究对象中，单纯腰围肥胖（OR = 1.57，95%CI：1.32 ~ 1.88）和单纯内脏肥胖（OR = 1.65，95%CI：1.33 ~ 2.05）同样是 10 年冠心病患病风险的危险因素。多项研究也证实腹型肥胖的人群糖尿病和冠心病患病率更高，腰围大于界值或是独立的慢性疾病的危险因素[19-22]。内脏型肥胖可显著增加冠心病发病风险[23]，更加精确地计算研究对象腹腔内脂肪含量，一定程度上弥补了单纯测量腰围的缺点。

综上所述，肥胖问题在新疆、西藏地区较为严重，男性、混合型肥胖（特别是 BMI 和腰围均异常）人群或是 10 年冠心病发病的高危人群。本研究具有一定的局限性，多因素分析中未调整饮食、体力活动、社会心理因素等混杂因素，故研究结果需要进一步验证。仅 BMI 肥胖人数少，可能因把握度有限而产生一定的偏倚。

致谢

感谢参与项目的所有专家及所有调查人员。协作组组成单位及主要调查人员：国家心血管病中心中国医学科学院阜外医院：王增武、张林峰、陈祚、王馨、邵澜、郭敏、田野、赵天明、范围辉、董莹、聂静雨、王佳丽、郑聪毅、贾秀云、朱曼璐、王文、陈伟伟、高润霖；卫生部北京医院：郭岩斐、孙铁英、王玉霞、柴迪、马雅立、仝亚琪；中国人民解放军总医院：陈韵岱、冯斌、朱庆磊、周珊珊、刘杰、王晶、杨丽娜、杨瑛、段鹏；新疆维吾尔自治区人民医院：李南方、周玲、张德莲、姚晓光、洪静、索菲亚、曹梅；中国疾病预防控制中心：吴静、石文惠、翟屹、何柳。

利益冲突

无。

参考文献

[1] Zhu KF, Wang YM. Zhu JZ. et al. National prevalence of coronary heart disease and its relationship with human development index: a systematic review [J]. Eur J Prev Cardiol, 2016, 23(5): 530-543. DOI: 10.1177/2047487315587402.

[2] 国家卫生和计划生育委员会. 中国卫生和计划生育统计年鉴 2015[M]. 北京：中国协和医科大学出版社.

[3] Wakabayashi I. Stronger associations of obesity with prehypertension and hypertension in young women than in young men [J]. J Hypertens, 2012, 30(7): 1423-1429. DOI: 10.1097/HJH. Ob013e3283544881.

[4] Wakabayashi I. Age-dependent influence of gender on the association between obesity and a cluster of cardiometabolic risk actors [J]. Gend Med, 2012, 9(4): 267-277. DOI: 10.1016/j. genm.2012.05.004.

[5] Gordon-Larsen P, Wang HJ, Popkin BM. Overweight dynamics in Chinese children and adults[J]. Obes Rev, 2014, 15(1): 37-48. DOI: lO. llll/obr.12121.

[6] 王增武，郝光，王馨，等. 我国中年人群超重 / 肥胖现况及心血管病危险因素聚集分析 [J]. 中华流行病学杂志，2014.35 (4): 354-358. DOI: 10.3760/cma. j. issn.0254-6450.2014.04.003.

[7] He J, Guo SX. Liu JM, et al. Ethnic differences in prevalence of general obesity and abdominal obesity among low-income rural Kazakh and Uyghur adults in far western China and implications in preventive public health [J]. PLoS One, 2014.9(9): e106723. DOI: 10.1371/journal. pone.0106723.

[8] Global Burden of Metabolic Risk Factors for Chronic Diseases Collaboration (BMI Mediated Effects), Lu Y, Hajifathalian K, et al. Metabolic mediators of the effects of body-mass index, overweight, and obesity on coronary heart disease and stroke: a pooled analysis of 97 prospective cohorts with 1.8 million participants [J]. Lancet, 2014, 383(9921): 970-983. DOI: 10.1016/s0140-6736(13)61836-x.

[9] Mongraw-Chaffin ML, Peters SA, Huxley RR, et al. The sex-specific association between BMI and coronary heart disease: a systematic review and Meta-analysis of 95 cohorts with 1.2 million participants [J]. Lancet Diabetes Endocrinol, 2015, 3(6): 437-449. DOI: 10.1016/s2213-8587(15)00086-8.

[10] Zhou BF. Cooperative Meta-analysis Group of the Working Group on Obesity in China. Predictive values of body mass index and waist circumference for risk factors of certain related diseases in Chinese adults-study on optimal cut-off points of body mass index and waist circumference in Chinese adults [J]. Biomed Environ Sci, 2002, 15(1): 83-96.

[11] 中国肥胖问题工作组. 中国成人超重和肥胖症预防与控制指南 (节录)[J]. 营养学报，2004, 26(1): 1-4.

DOI: 10.3321/j issn.0512-7955.2004.01.001.

[12] 诸骏仁，高润霖，赵水平，等. 中国成人血脂异常防治指南 (2016 年修订版)[J]. 中国循环杂志，2016, 31(10): 937-953. DOI: 10.3969/j. issn.1000-3614.2016.10.001.

[13] Examination Committee of Criteria for 'Obesity Disease' in Japan, Japan Society for the Study of Obesity. New criteria for 'obesity disease' in Japan [J]. Circ J, 2002.66(11): 987-992.

[14] Liu J, Hong Y, D 'Agostino RB Sr, et al. Predictive value for the Chinese population of the Framingham CHD risk assessment tool compared with the Chinese Multi-Provincial Cohort Study [J]. JAMA, 2004, 291(21): 2591-2599. DOI: 10.1001/jama.291.21.2591.

[15] 王玉林，张丽，何佳，等. 新疆偏远农村地区成年人血压与肥胖指标的关系 [J]. 中华高血压杂志，2016.24(7): 650-656. DOI: 10.16439/j. cnki.1673-7245.2016.07.013.

[16] Zhang P, Wang R, Gao CS, et al. Types of obesity and its association with the clustering of cardiovascular disease risk factors in Jilin province of China [J]. Int J Environ Res Public Health, 2016, 13(7): 685. DOI: 10.3390/ijerph13070685.

[17] Jiang JC, Deng SY, Chen Y, et al. Comparison of visceral and body fat indices and anthropometric measures in relation to untreated hypertension by age and gender among Chinese [J]. Int J Cardio1, 2016, 219: 204-211. DOI: 10.1016/j. ijcard.2016.06.032.

[18] 刘晨，张黎军. 新型体脂指数和内脏脂肪指数的相关研究进展 [J]. 中国糖尿病杂志，2016(ll): 1032-1035. DOI: 10.3969/j. issn.1006-6187.2016.11.16.

[19] Velasquez-Rodriguez CM, Velasquez-Villa M, Gomez-Ocampo L. et al. Abdominal obesity and low physical activity are associated with insulin resistance in overweight adolescents: a cross-sectional study [J]. BMC Pediatr, 2014, 14: 258. DOI: 10.1186/1471-2431-14-258.

[20] Garcia-Hermoso A, Martinez-Vizcaino V, Recio-Rodriguez JI, et al. Abdominal obesity as a mediator of the influence of physical activity on insulin resistance in Spanish adults [J]. Prev Med, 2016, 82: 59-64. DOI: 10.1016/j. ypmed.2015.11.012.

[21] Rheaume C, Arsenault BJ, Despres JP, et al. Impact of abdominal obesity and systemic hypertension on risk of coronary heart disease in men and women: the EPIC-Norfolk Population Study [J]. J Hypertens, 2014, 32(11): 2224-2230. DOI: 10.1097/hjh.0000000000000307.

[22] Canoy D, Caims BJ, Balkwill A, et al. Coronary heart disease incidence in women by waist circumference within categories of body mass index [J]. Eur J Prev Cardiol, 2013, 20(5): 759-762. DOI: 10.1177/2047487313492631.

[23] Zhang XL, Shu XO, Li HL, et al. Visceral adiposity and risk of coronary heart disease in relatively lean Chinese adults [J]. Int J Cardiol, 2013, 168(3): 2141-2145. DOI: 10.1016/j. ijcard.2013.01.275.

新疆和西藏地区居民体重指数及腰围与10年冠状动脉粥样硬化性心脏病发病风险的关系△

郑聪毅，王增武，陈 祚，张林峰，王 馨，董 莹，聂静雨，王佳丽，邵 澜，田 野

中国医学科学院阜外医院，国家心血管病中心社区防治部 北京．102308

通讯作者：王增武，E-mail：wangzengwu@foxmail.com

摘 要 目的 探讨我国新疆和西藏地区居民体重指数、腰围与10年冠状动脉粥样硬化性心脏病（冠心病）发病风险的关系。**方法** 采用多阶段分层随机抽样的方法，于2015年6月至2017年3月共抽取新疆和西藏地区≥35岁研究对象7 631例，其中资料完整的5 737例纳入分析。体重指数分为3个等级组：A组＜24 kg/m²（2 005例）、B组24～＜28 kg/m²（2 178例）、C组≥28 kg/m²（1 554例）。腰围分为3个等级组：Ⅰ组＜85（男）/80（女）cm（1 657例）、Ⅱ组85～＜90（男）/80～＜85（女）cm（973例）、Ⅲ组≥90（男）/85（女）cm（3 107例）。应用中国多省队列研究（CMCS）10年冠心病发病风险预测模型，探究体重指数及腰围与冠心病发病风险的关系。**结果** 体重指数C组和腰围Ⅲ组高血压、高总胆固醇、低HDL-C和糖尿病比例较大（均$P<0.01$）。体重指数各等级组的10年冠心病发病风险绝对值随腰围水平的增加而增加（趋势检验$P<0.000\ 1$）；对于腰围水平低的对象，其体重指数水平越高，冠心病发病风险绝对值越高（趋势检验$P=0.000\ 6$）。多因素Logistic分析显示，对于同一体重指数（或腰围）等级的研究对象，其10年冠心病发病风险随腰围（或体重指数）水平的增加而增加（趋势检验$P<0.05$）；体重指数C组且腰围Ⅲ组的冠心病发病风险最大（比值＝4.191，95%置信区间：3.578～4.909）。**结论** 新疆和西藏地区居民体重指数和腰围是10年冠心病发病风险的独立影响因素，体重指数和腰围同时处于较高水平者或是10年冠心病发病的高危人群。

关键词 冠状动脉粥样硬化性心脏病；体重指数；腰围；发病风险

△ 本文发表于：中国医药，2017，12（7）：965-970.

Association among Body Mass Index, Waist Circumference and 10-year Coronary Atherosclerotic Heart Disease in Xinjiang and Tibet Regions of China

Zheng Congyi, Wang Zengwu, Chen Zuo, Zhang Linfeng, Wang Xin, Dong Ying, Nie Jingye, Wang Jiali, Shao Lan, Tian Ye

Department of Prevention and Community Health, National Center For Cardiovascular Diseases, Fuwai Hospital, Chinese Academy of Medical Sciences, Beijing 102308

Corresponding author: Wang Zengwu, Email: wangzengwu@foxmail. com

Abstract **Objective** To investigate the association among body mass index (BMI), waist circumference (WC) and the 10-year coronary atherosclerotic heart disease (CHD) in Xinjiang and Tibet areas of China. **Methods** Based on stratified multi-stage random sampling method, 7, 631people of 35 years or older were enrolled from Xinjiang and Tibet regions from June 2015 to March 2017; 5, 737cases with complete data were analyzed. BMI and WC were measured; the population was allocated into group A [BMI < 24 kg/m^2(2, 005 cases)], group B [BMI 24– < 28 kg/m^2 (2, 178 cases)], and group C [BMI ≥ 28 kg/m^2 (1, 554cases)]; group Ⅰ [WC < 85 cm (males)/80 cm (females) (1 657cases)], group Ⅱ [WC85– < 90 cm (males)/80– < 85 cm (females) (973 cases)], and group Ⅲ (WC ≥ 90 cm (males)/ > 85 cm (females) (3107cases). The relation among BMI, WC and CHD risk were analyzed based on the Chinese Multi-provincial Cohort Study (CMCS) 10-year CHD risk prediction model. **Results** Group C and group Ⅲ had higher percentages of hypertension, high total cholesterol, lower high-density lipoprotein cholesterol and diabetes compared to the groups with lower BMI or WC($P < 0.01$). The absolute 10-year CHD risk increased with WC in groups with same BMI ($P < 0.000\ 1$); it increased with BMI in population with low WC($P < 0.000\ 6$). Multivariate Logistic analysis showed that 10-year CHD risk increased with BMI(or WC)in groups with same WC(or BMI) ($P < 0.05$); group C + group Ⅲ had the highest 10-year CHD risk (odds ratio = 4.191, 95% confidence interval: 3.578 – 4.909). **Conclusions** Both BMI and WC are independently associated with the 10-year CHD risk; the population with higher BMI and WC has a higher 10-year CHD risk in Tibet and Xinjiang areas of China.

Key words Coronary atherosclerotic heart disease; Body mass index; Waist circumference; Risk

冠状动脉粥样硬化性心脏病（冠心病）和脑卒中是全球首要死因[1]。在发展中国家，冠心病患病率与国家发展指数呈正比[2]。2002 ~ 2014 年中国冠心病病死率呈上升趋势，2014 年我国城市冠心病病死率为 107.5/10 万，农村为 105.37/10 万[3]。随着经济发展和生活方式的变化，肥胖患病率持续上升，已成为心血管疾病的重要危险因素[4]。肥胖可增加 0.5 ~ 1.0 倍冠心病发病风险，且近 23% 的冠心病是由肥胖引起的[5, 6]。我国新疆地区人群肥胖或腹型肥胖的患病率明显高于全国平均水平[7]，但西藏地区居民肥胖情况少有全面系统的报道。本研究利用公益性行业科研专项“西藏与新疆地区慢性心肺疾病现状调查研究”的相关数据，中国多省队列研究（CMCS）中 Framingham 校正后预测模型[8]评估新疆和西藏地区居民的 10 年冠心病发病风险，并探讨体重指数和腰围与 10 年冠心病发病风险的关系，为制定我国西部地区有效预防和控制冠心病等心血管疾病策略提供科学依据。

1. 对象与方法

1.1 对象

本研究是公益性行业科研专项“西藏与新疆地区慢性心肺疾病现状调查研究”的一部分。该项目于 2015 年 6 月至 2017 年 3 月在我国新疆和西藏地区采用分层 4 阶段随机抽样方法抽取调查对象。首先分别在新疆和西藏自治区内按城乡分为 2 层，每层内采用与容量大小成比例的概率抽取所需数量的区 / 县；然后在被抽中的区 / 县中采用简单随机抽样（SRS）方法抽取 2 个街道 / 乡镇；再在被抽中的街道 / 乡镇中采用 SRS 方法抽取 3 个居委会 / 村委会；最后在被抽中的居委会 / 村委会中分性别、年龄采用 SRS 方法抽取调查个体。该项目在新疆抽取 7 个区 / 县，在西藏抽取 6 个区 / 县，每个区 / 县样本量为 15 岁及以上对象 1 000 人。本研究实际入选 35 岁及以上调查对象 7 631 例，其中资料完整的 5 737 例数据纳入分析。

1.2 研究方法

1.2.1 问卷调查和体格检查　调查对象采用统一的调查方案、调查手册及调查问卷。主要参与调查人员均进行培训并通过考核。问卷内容包括一般人口学特征、生活方式和行为、个人疾病史及家族史。血压的测量采用日本欧姆龙 HBP-1300 电子血压计，每位对象静坐 5 min 后测血压，取连续 3 次（每次至少间隔 30 秒）读数的平均值为个体血压值，测量前 30 分钟内避免吸烟、饮酒、饮用含有咖啡因的饮料及剧烈运动。体质量的测量采用日本欧姆龙 V-BODY HBF.37 1 体质量体脂测量仪。

1.2.2 实验室检测　每位调查对象采集空腹 12 小时外周静脉血标本，测定空腹血糖、血脂 [三酰甘油、总胆固醇、高密度脂蛋白胆固醇（HDL-C）、低密度脂蛋白胆固醇（LDL-C）] 等。标本先保存于 − 70℃冰箱，所有标本采集完成后统一检测。生化指标测定采用日本 Hitachi 7080 型自动生化分析仪。血糖水平通过葡萄糖氧化酶过氧化物酶偶联体系方法测定，血脂指标通过酶法测定。

1.2.3 质量控制　现场调查前，本项目组成员对各地区调查骨干和人员进行严格培训和考核，并进行为期 1 周左右的现场督导；为确保各环节的质量，调查现场设有固定的质量控制人员；为确保调查数据和体格检查数据的质量，统一采用现场Pad录入并随时上传数据，调查数据及时核查和反馈。

1.3 分组标准及定义

1.3.1 肥胖指标　根据《中国成人超重与肥胖症预防与控制指南（节录）》[9]超重和肥胖的切点值，将研究对象按体重指数分为3个等级组：A组 < 24 kg/m^2（2 005例）、B组24 ~ < 28 kg/m^2（2 178例）、C组≥ 28 kg/m^2（1 554例）。结合本研究中男性和女性腰围均值（90 cm、87 cm）和标准差（0.5-SD近5 cm）以及《中国成人血脂异常防治指南（2016年修订版）》[10]腹型肥胖的界值，将研究对象按腰围分为3个等级组：Ⅰ组 < 85（男）/80（女）cm（1 657例）、Ⅱ组85 ~ < 90（男）/80 ~ < 85（女）cm（973例）、Ⅲ组≥ 90（男）/85（女）cm（3 107例）。

1.3.2 10年冠心病发病风险预测模型　CMCS10年冠心病发病风险预测模型[8]中包括年龄、血压、总胆固醇、HDL-C、吸烟、糖尿病6项指标。①血压等级：理想血压 < 120/80 mmHg、正常血压120 ~ < 130/80 ~ < 85 mmHg、正常高值130 ~ < 140/85 ~ < 90 mmHg、Ⅰ级高血压140 ~ < 160/90 ~ < 100 mmHg、Ⅱ级及以上高血压≥ 160/100 mmHg，如果收缩压和舒张压分别在不同等级则取最高等级；②总胆固醇等级：< 160、160 ~ < 200、200 ~ < 240、240 ~ < 280、≥ 280 mg/dl；③HDL-C等级：< 35、35 ~ < 45、45 ~ < 50、50 ~ < 60、≥ 60 mg/dl；④吸烟定义为至少吸过20包且最近1个月仍在吸烟；⑤糖尿病定义为既往确诊或实验室检查非同日2次或以上空腹血糖≥ 7.0 mmol/L。

1.4 统计学分析

采用SAS 9.3统计软件进行数据处理。计量资料以$\bar{x}$ ± SD表示，组间比较采用两独立样本t检验或单因素方差分析，两两比较采用SNK法；计数资料组间比较用χ^2检验；等级资料比较采用Kruskal-Wallis秩和检验。均值或比值比的趋势性检验采用广义线性模型计算趋势P值。多因素分析采用多元Logistic回归，采用有序多分类响应变量Logistic回归；由于自然人群中的10年冠心病发病风险大多集中在 < 5%，故本研究多因素Logistic分析中采用四分位法对冠心病发病风险进行等级处理。P < 0.05为差异有统计学意义。

2. 结果

2.1 一般情况

5 737例研究对象的基本信息统计结果见表1。不同性别比较，男性的汉族、初中及以上学历、吸烟、饮酒比例、舒张压、三酰甘油、空腹血糖、腰围水平明显高于女性；女性高居住地海拔、总胆固醇、HDL-C、BMI 水平明显高于男性（均 $P < 0.05$）。

表 1　新疆和西藏地区 5 737 例研究对象的基本特征

项　　目	男性（$n = 2\,526$）	女性（$n = 3\,211$）	合　　计
年龄（岁，$\bar{x} \pm SD$）	53.4 ± 13.0	52.9 ± 12.3	53.1 ± 12.6
汉族 [例（%）][a]	1 085（43.0）	1 005（31.3）	2 090（36.4）
农村户口 [例（%）]	1 905（75.4）	2 427（75.6）	4 332（75.5）
初中及以上学历 [例（%）][a]	1 056（41.8）	975（30.4）	2 031（35.4）
居住地海拔 [米，例（%）][a]			
＜1 000	1 282（50.8）	1 394（43.4）	2 676（46.6）
1 000～＜3 500	871（34.5）	1 065（33.2）	1 936（33.7）
≥3 500	373（14.8）	752（23.4）	1 125（19.6）
吸烟 [例（%）][a]	1 098（43.5）	120（3.7）	1 218（21.2）
饮酒 [例（%）][a]	1 123（44.5）	466（14.5）	1 589（27.7）
收缩压（mmHg，$\bar{x} \pm SD$）	131.1 ± 19.9	130.8 ± 22.1	13.9 ± 21.2
舒张压（mmHg，$\bar{x} \pm SD$）[a]	79.8 ± 12.1	77.2 ± 12.1	78.4 ± 12.2
三酰甘油（mg/dl，$\bar{x} \pm SD$）[a]	119.3 ± 86.0	98.4 ± 57.3	107.7 ± 72.3
总胆固醇（mg/dl，$\bar{x} \pm SD$）[b]	179.2 ± 35.3	181.5 ± 37.0	180.4 ± 36.3
HDL-C（mg/dl，$\bar{x} \pm SD$）[a]	51.8 ± 11.7	58.1 ± 11.9	55.4 ± 12.2
LDL-C（mg/dl，$\bar{x} \pm SD$）	105.8 ± 29.3	105.2 ± 30.3	105.5 ± 29.9
空腹血糖（mmol/L，$\bar{x} \pm SD$）[a]	5.4 ± 1.7	5.1 ± 1.4	5.2 ± 1.5
体重指数（kg/m^2，$\bar{x} \pm SD$）[b]	25.4 ± 3.7	25.7 ± 4.1	25.6 ± 3.9
腰围（cm，$\bar{x} \pm SD$）[a]	89.9 ± 10.7	86.7 ± 11.5	88.1 ± 11.2

注：吸烟定义为至少吸过 20 包且最近 1 个月仍在吸烟；饮酒定义为最近 1 个月每周至少饮酒 1 次；HDL-C 为高密度脂蛋白胆固醇；LDL-C 为低密度脂蛋白胆固醇；男性与女性比较，a. $P < 0.01$，b. $P < 0.05$。

2.2　不同体重指数和腰围水平研究对象

10 年冠心病预测模型变量和发病风险绝对值情况体重指数 C 组和腰围Ⅲ组高血压、高总胆固醇、低 HDL-C 和糖尿病比例较大（均 $P < 0.01$）（表 2、表 3）。体重指数各等级组的

冠心病发病风险绝对值随腰围水平的增加而增加（趋势检验 $P < 0.0001$）；对于腰围水平低的对象，其体重指数水平越高，冠心病发病风险绝对值越高（趋势检验 $P = 0.0006$），见表 4。

表 2　新疆和西藏地区不同体重指数水平研究对象的冠心病危险因素分析

危险因素	A 组（$n = 2005$）	B 组（$n = 2178$）	C 组（$n = 1554$）
男性 [例（%）][a]	861（42.9）	1 011（46.4）	654（42.1）
年龄（岁，$\bar{x} \pm SD$）[b]	53.2 ± 13.5	52.5 ± 12.3	53.5 ± 11.8[c]
吸烟 [例（%）][b]	481（24.0）	451（20.7）	286（18.4）
糖尿病 [例（%）][b]	70（3.5）	147（6.7）	155（10.0）
血压 [mmHg，例（%）][b]			
＜120/80	904（45.1）	658（30.2）	248（16.0）
120～＜130/80～＜85	382（19.0）	478（22.0）	313（20.1）
130～＜140/85～＜90	264（13.2）	382（17.5）	297（19.1）
140～＜160/90～＜100	267（13.3）	414（19.0）	419（27.0）
≥ 160/100	188（9.4）	246（11.3）	277（17.8）
总胆固醇 [mg/dl，例（%）][b]			
＜160	713（35.6）	601（27.6）	362（23.3）
160～＜200	847（42.2）	938（43.1）	688（44.3）
200～＜240	357（17.8）	507（23.3）	393（25.3）
240～＜280	69（3.4）	110（5.0）	92（5.9）
≥ 280	19（0.9）	22（1.0）	19（1.2）
HDL-C[mg/dl，例（%）][b]			
＜35	30（1.5）	37（1.7）	43（2.8）
35～＜45	237（11.8）	423（19.4）	316（20.3）
45～＜50	265（13.2）	357（16.4）	290（18.7）
50～＜60	604（30.1）	721（33.1）	511（32.9）
≥ 60	869（43.3）	640（29.4）	394（25.4）

注：A 组体重指数 ＜ 24 kg/m^2；B 组体重指数 24～＜ 28 kg/m^2；C 组体重指数≥ 28 kg/m^2；冠心病为冠状动脉粥样硬化性心脏病；HDL-C 为高密度脂蛋白胆固醇；A、B、C 3 组间比较，[a] $P < 0.05$、[b] $P < 0.01$；与 A、B 组比较，[c] $P < 0.05$。

表 3　新疆和西藏地区不同腰围水平研究对象的冠心病危险因素分析

危险因素	Ⅰ组（n＝1 657）	Ⅱ组（n＝973）	Ⅲ组（n＝3 107）
男性［例（%）］[a]	769（46.4）	449（46.1）	1 308（42.1）
年龄（岁，$\bar{x} \pm SD$）[a]	52.2 ± 13.1	52.5 ± 12.5	53.8 ± 12.4[b]
吸烟［例（%）］[a]	416（25.1）	223（22.9）	579（18.6）
糖尿病［例（%）］[a]	50（3.0）	42（4.3）	180（9.0）
血压［mmHg，例（%）］[a]			
＜120/80	778（47.0）	338（34.7）	694（22.3）
120～＜130/80～＜85	324（19.6）	216（22.2）	633（20.4）
130～＜140/85～＜90	216（13.0）	160（16.4）	567（18.2）
140～＜160/90～＜100	190（11.5）	160（16.4）	750（24.1）
≥160/100	149（9.0）	99（10.2）	463（14.9）
总胆固醇［mg/dl，例（%）］[a]			
＜160	622（37.5）	278（28.6）	776（2.0）
160～＜200	733（44.2）	412（42.3）	1 328（42.7）
200～＜240	249（15.0）	227（23.3）	781（25.1）
240～＜280	42（2.5）	41（4.2）	188（6.1）
≥280	11（0.7）	15（1.5）	34（1.1）
HDL-C［mg/dl，例（%）］[a]			
＜35	26（1.6）	17（1.7）	67（2.2）
35～＜45	194（11.7）	147（15.1）	635（20.4）
45～＜50	222（13.4）	143（14.7）	547（17.6）
50～＜60	513（31.0）	320（32.9）	1 003（32.3）
≥60	702（42.4）	346（35.6）	855（27.5）

注：Ⅰ组膜围＜85（男）/80（女）cm；Ⅱ组腰围85～＜90（男）/80～＜85（女）cm；m组腰围≥90（男）/85（女）cm；冠心病为冠状动脉粥样硬化性心脏病；HDL-C为高密度脂蛋白胆固醇；Ⅰ、Ⅱ、Ⅲ 3组间比较，[a]$P < 0.01$；与Ⅰ、Ⅱ组比较，[b]均$P < 0.05$。

表 4　新疆和西藏地区不同体重指数和腰围水平研究对象
10 年冠心病发病风险绝对值比较 [例数，M (P_{25}，P_{75})，%]

组　别	Ⅰ组	Ⅱ组	Ⅲ组	趋势 P 值
男性				
A 组	634, 1.07（0.55, 2.10）	142, 1.27（0.67, 2.53）	85, 1.74（0.89, 3.08）	>0.05
B 组	127, 0.94（0.54, 1.81）	277, 1.18（0.64, 2.14）	607, 1.48（0.77, 2.68）	<0.000 1
C 组	8, 0.87（0.61, 1.79）	30, 1.44（0.78, 2.58）	616, 1.50（0.79, 2.96）	>0.05
趋势 P 值	0.006 7	>0.05	>0.05	
女性				
A 组	737, 0.31（0.14, 0.85）	239, 0.50（0.19, 1.38）	168, 0.70（0.25, 2.43）	<0.000 1
B 组	136, 0.36（0.20, 0.68）	259, 0.44（0.21, 1.10）	772, 0.64（0.29, 1.71）	<0.000 1
C 组	15, 0.42（0.31, 1.11）	26, 0.54（0.36, 1.14）	859, 0.86（0.39, 2.01）	<0.000 1
趋势 P 值	0.015 1	>0.05	>0.05	
合计				
A 组	1 371, 0.49（0.32, 1.20）	381, 0.78（0.31, 1.84）	253, 1.08（0.39, 2.79）	<0.000 1
B 组	263, 0.56（0.29, 1.23）	536, 0.80（0.35, 1.78）	1 379, 1.00（0.40, 2.29）	<0.000 1
C 组	23, 0.62（0.26, 1.54）	56, 1.05（0.46, 2.19）	1 475, 1.11（0.53, 2.48）	<0.000 1
趋势 P 值	0.000 6	>0.05	>0.05	

注：A 组体重指数 <24 kg/m^2；B 组体重指数 24～<28 kg/m^2；C 组体重指数≥28 kg/m^2；Ⅰ组腰围 <85（男）/80（女）cm；Ⅱ组腰围 85～<90（男）/80～<85（女）cm；Ⅲ组腰围≥90（男）/85（女）cm；冠心病为冠状动脉粥样硬化性心脏病。

2.3　体重指数及腰围与 10 年冠心病发病风险的关系

以 10 年冠心病发病风险四分位等级变量作因变量进行多因素 Logistic 分析。调整了性别、年龄、民族、饮酒、居住地海拔、受教育程度、农村 / 城镇户口、冠心病家族史 8 个 10 年冠心病风险预测模型之外的混杂因素，结果表明，与体重指数 A 组且腰围Ⅰ组的研究对象比较，体重指数 C 组且腰围Ⅱ组、体重指数 B 组且腰围Ⅲ组的冠心病发病风险明显增加；体重指数 C 组且腰围Ⅲ组的发病风险最大。对于同一体重指数 A、B、C 组（或腰围Ⅱ、Ⅲ组）等级的研究对象，其 10 年冠心病发病风险随腰围（或体重指数）水平的增加而呈增加趋势（趋势检验 $P<0.05$），见表 5。

表 5　新疆和西藏地区不同体重指数和腰围水平研究对象
10 年冠心病发病风险多因素 Logistic 分析 [比值比（95% 置信区间）]

组　别	Ⅰ组	Ⅱ组	Ⅲ组	趋势 P 值
A 组	1.000	1.603（1.268 ~ 2.026）	1.584（1.190 ~ 2.106）	< 0.000 1
B 组	1.444（1.106 ~ 1.886）	1.799（1.463 ~ 2.211）	2.769（2.365 ~ 3.241）	< 0.000 1
C 组	1.278（0.560 ~ 2.914）	2.236（1.287 ~ 3.886）	4.191（3.578 ~ 4.909）	0.000 6
趋势 P 值	0.287 0	0.014 9	< 0.000 1	

注：A 组体重指数 < 24 kg/m^2；B 组体重指数 24 ~ < 28 kg/m^2；C 组体重指数≥ 28 kg/m^2；Ⅰ组腰围 < 85（男）/80（女）cm；Ⅱ组腰围 85 ~ < 90（男）/80 ~ < 85（女）cm；Ⅲ组腰围≥ 90（男）/85（女）cm；冠心病为冠状动脉粥样硬化性心脏病。

3. 讨论

前瞻性研究表明体重指数、腰围等肥胖指标与冠心病发病密切相关[11，12]。新疆和西藏地区≥ 35 岁人群体重指数和腰围水平高于全国中年人，可能是因为新疆和西藏地区居民高脂肪、高热量、高盐的独特饮食方式以及独特的自然环境、文化生活方式等导致肥胖诱导因素以及心血管疾病危险因素聚集[13]，故探究新疆和西藏地区居民的肥胖指标与冠心病发病风险更有公共卫生学意义。

本研究发现，对于同一体重指数（或腰围）等级的研究对象，其 10 年冠心病发病风险随腰围（或体重指数）水平的增加呈增加趋势（$P < 0.05$），高水平体重指数和腰围或是 10 年冠心病发病风险的独立危险因素。英国一项大型队列研究对近 50 万中年女性进行了 5 年随访，结果表明体重指数和腰围均是冠心病的独立危险因素，相同体重指数（或腰围）等级组的调整发病率随腰围（或体重指数）水平的增加而增加[14]。Wormser 等[15]汇总 17 个国家 58 项大型前瞻性研究结果表明，应用体重指数、腰围和腰臀预测心血管疾病时，单一指标或结合多项肥胖指标预测能力相当，特别是结合收缩压、糖尿病家族史和血脂情况下；但结合体重指数和腰围可以更好地反应研究对象的三酰甘油和 HDL-C 水平，进而更好地预测心血管疾病或其他慢性疾病[9]。其原因可能是，一方面体重指数和腰围有各自的优点，体重指数可以判断整体肥胖情况，腰围可以较好反映内脏脂肪累积程度，是糖尿病和心血管疾病的独立危险因素[16]，二者某种程度上在预测冠心病发病风险中具有加和作用；另一方面，将体重指数和腰围结合分析，弥补了各自的缺点，如体重指数仅考虑体质量而忽略了成分，无法区分体内瘦组织和脂肪组织所占的比例[17]，而腰围受身高影响且无法区分皮下和内脏脂肪，且忽略了身高的影响。

然而，在冠心病等心血管疾病的预测中，血压、血脂和血糖等指标比体重指数、腰围等肥胖指标能力更强且更精准，因而是包括本研究所用预测模型在内的类似预测模型的重要变量。但体重指数和腰围测量方便而经济，且对10年冠心病发病风险具有较好的预测价值，故对于我国新疆和西藏地区冠心病等心血管疾病高危人群初筛中更有实际价值，体重指数和腰围水平均较高人群应为冠心病等心血管疾病预防和控制的重点干预对象。但在重点人群干预过程中不容忽视的是，一味追求将肥胖指标水平下降到正常值而不符合临床基本原则可能适得其反，有干预性研究结果显示，体质量短时间变化（增加或减少）幅度过大是冠心病发病的危险因素[18]。

综上，新疆和西藏地区居民体重指数和腰围水平高是10年冠心病发病风险的危险因素，体重指数和腰围同时处于较高水平者或是10年冠心病发病的高危人群。本研究具有一定的局限性，横断面研究结论需进一步前瞻性或干预性研究证实；多因素分析中未调整体力活动、饮食、社会心理因素等混杂因素；统计表中部分格子频数过低，可能导致检验效能和方向上的偏倚，故本研究结果需要进一步验证。

致谢

感谢参与项目的所有专家及调查人员。协作组组成单位及主要调查人员：国家心血管病中心、中国医学科学院阜外医院：郭敏、赵天明、范国辉、贾秀云、朱曼璐、王文、陈伟伟、高润霖；北京医院：郭岩斐、孙铁英、王玉霞、柴迪、马雅立、仝亚琪；解放军总医院：陈韵岱、冯斌、朱庆磊、周珊珊、刘杰、王晶、杨丽娜、杨瑛、段鹏；新疆维吾尔自治区人民医院：李南方、周玲、张德莲、姚晓光、洪静、索菲亚、曹梅；中国疾病预防控制中心：吴静、石文惠、翟屹、何柳。

参考文献

[1] Lozano R, Naghavi M, Foreman K, et al. Global and regional mortality from 235 causes of death for 20 age groups in 1990 and 2010: a systematic analysis for the Global Burden of Disease Study 2010 [J]. Lancet, 2012, 380(9859): 2095-2128. DOI: 10. 1016/s0140-6736(12)61728-0.

[2] Zhu KF, Wang YM, Z JZ, et al. National prevalence of coronary heart disease and its relationship with human development index: A systematic review [J]. Eur J Prev Cardiol, 2016, 23(5): 530-543. DOI: 10. 117/2047487315587402.

[3] 国家卫生和计划生育委员会．中国卫生和计划生育统计年鉴 2015[R]．北京：中国协和医科大学出版社，2015: 286-302.

[4] Lu J, Bi Y, Wang T, et al. The relationship between insulin-sensitive obesity and cardiovascular diseases in a Chinese population: results of the REACTION study [J]. Int J Cardiol, 2014, 172(2): 388-394. DOI: 10. 1016/j. ijcard. 2014. 01. 073.

[5] Mongraw-Chaffin ML, Peters SA, Huxley RR, et al. The sex-specific association between BMI and coronary heart disease: a systematic review and meta-analysis of 95 cohorts with 1. 2 million participants [J]. Lancet Diabetes Endocrinol, 2015, 3(6): 437-449. DOI: 10. 1016/s2213-8587(15)00086-8.

[6]Global Burden of Metabolic Risk Factors for Chronic Diseases Collaboration (BMI Mediated Effects), Lu Y, Hajifathalian K, et al. Metabolic mediators of the effects of body-mass index, overweight, and obesity on coronary heart disease and stroke: a pooled analysis of 97 prospective cohorts with 1. 8 million participants [J]. Lancet, 2014, 383(9921): 970-983. DOI: 10. 1016/s0140-6736(13)61836-x.

[7] He J, Guo S, Liu J, et al. Ethnic differences in prevalence of general obesity and abdominal obesity among low-income rural Kazakh an Uyghur adults in far western China and implications in preventive public health [J]. PloS One, 2014, 9(9): e106723. DOI: 10. 1371/journal. pone. 0106723.

[8] Liu J, Hong Y, D'Agostino RB Sr, et al. Predictive value for the Chinese population of the Framingham CHD risk assessment tool compared with the Chinese Multi-Provincial Cohort Study [J]. JAMA, 2004, 291(21): 2591-2599. DOI: 10. 1001/jama. 291. 21. 2591.

[9] 中国肥胖问题工作组 . 中国成人超重与肥胖症预防与控制指南 (节录)[J]. 营养学报 , 2004, 26(1): 1-4. DOI: 10. 13325/j. cnki. acta. nutr. sin. 2004. 01. 001.

[10] 中国成人血脂异常防治指南修订联合委员会．中国成人血脂异常防治指南 (2016 年修订版)[J]．中国循环杂志，2017, 16(1): 937-953. DOI: 10. 3760/cma. j. issn. 1671-7368. 2017. 01. 006.

[11] Stegger JG, Schmidt EB, Obel T, et al. Body composition and body fat distribution in relation to later risk of acute myocardial infarction: a Danish follow-up study [J]. Int J Obes (Lond), 2011, 35(11): 1433-1441. DOI: 10. 1038/ijo. 2010. 278.

[12] Wildman RP, McGinn AP, Lin J, et al. Cardiovascular disease risk of abdominal obesity vs. metabolic abnormalities [J]. Obesity (Silver Spring), 2011, 19(4): 853-860. DOI: 10. 1038/oby. 2010. 168.

[13] 王玉林，张丽，何佳，等．新疆偏远农村地区成年人血压与肥胖指标的关系 [J]．中华高血压杂志，2016, 24(7): 650-656. DOI: 10. 16439/j. cnki. 1673-7245. 2016. 07. 013.

[14] Canoy D, Cairns BJ, Balkwill A, et al. Coronary heart disease incidence in women by waist circumference within categories of body mass index [J]. Eur J Prev Cardiol, 2013, 20(5): 759-762. DOI: 10. 1177/2047487313492631.

[15] Emerging Risk Factors Collaboration, Wormser D, Kaptoge S, et al. Separate and combined associations of body-mass index and abdominal adiposity with cardiovascular disease: collaborative analysis of 58 prospective studies [J]. Lancet, 2011, 377(9771): 1085-1095. DOI: 10. 1016/s0140-6736(11)60105-0.

[16] Garcia-Hermoso A, Martinez-Vizcaino V, Recio-Rodriguez Ji, et al. Abdoninal obesity as a mediator of the influence of physical activity on insulin resistance in Spanish adults [J]. Prev Med, 2016(82): 59-64. DOI: 10. 1016/j. ypmed. 2015. 11. 012.

[17] Jiang J, Deng S, Chen Y, et al. Comparison of visceral and body fat indices and anthropometric measures in relation to untreated hypertension by age and gender among Chinese [J]. Int J Cardiol, 2016(219): 204-211. DOI: 10. 1016/j. ijcard. 2016. 06. 032.

[18] Stevenis J, Erber E, Truesdale KP, et al. Long-and short-term weight change and incident coronary heart disease and ischemic stroke: the Atherosclerosis Risk in Communities Study [J]. Am J Epidemiol, 2013, 178(2): 239-248. DOI: 10. 1093/aje/kws461.

新疆地区居民代谢健康型肥胖的患病率及影响因素△

王佳丽，陈　祚，张林峰，王　馨，董　莹，聂静雨，郑聪毅，邵　澜，田　野，王增武

中国医学科学院阜外医院，国家心血管病中心社区防治部　北京 . 102308
通讯作者：王增武，E-mail：wangzengwu@foxmail.com

摘　要　目的　探讨新疆地区居民代谢健康型肥胖（metabolic healthy obesity，MHO）的患病率及影响因素。**方法**　2015 年至 2016 年期间，采用分层多阶段随机抽样，选取新疆地区 35 ~ 80 岁调查对象 4 627 人，有效数据 3 456 人（74.69%）。肥胖和代谢状态分类基于体重指数（BMI）和代谢异常组分的数量。**结果**　调查人群中 MHO 患病率为 16.09%，肥胖人群 MHO 患病率为 59.15%。女性中 MHO 比例随着年龄增加而下降（$P < 0.01$），男性中未见该趋势（$P > 0.05$）。农村居民 MHO 比例显著高于城市（64.75% vs.43.27%，$P < 0.01$）。汉族（OR = 0.33，95%CI：0.23 ~ 0.45）、腰围（WC）增加（每 5 cm）（OR = 0.80，95%CI：0.73 ~ 0.88）与 MHO 患病风险下降相关，中度职业体力劳动（OR = 2.92，95%CI：1.75 ~ 4.88）与 MHO 患病风险增加相关。调整内脏脂肪指数（VFI）模型中，VFI 升高（OR = 0.80，95%CI：0.73 ~ 0.88）与 MHO 患病风险下降相关。**结论**　新疆地区 35 ~ 80 岁居民 MHO 患病率较高。年龄、民族、中度职业劳动强度、WC 和 VFI 与肥胖人群的代谢状态有关。

关键词　代谢；肥胖；患病率；危险因素；新疆地区

Prevalence and Determinants of Metabolic Healthy Obesity in Xinjiang Population

Wang Jiali, Chen Zuo, Zhang Linfeng, Wang Xin, Dong Ying, Nie Jing yu, Zheng Cong yi, Shao Lan, Tian Ye, Wang Zeng wu

Fuwai Hospital, Chinese Academy of Medical Sciences, Beijing 102308, China

△　本文发表于：心血管病防治，2017，7（3）：164-168.

Abstract **Objective** To investigate the prevalence of metabolic healthy obesity (MHO) in Xinjiang population and to identify the determinants related to MHO. **Methods** Using stratified multi-stage random sampling, a total of 4 627 residents aged 35 – 80 years were examined with international standardized examination in 2015-2016. At length, 3 456 participants were eligible for analysis. The obesity and metabolic status were classified based on body mass index (BMI) and the number of abnormalities in components of metabolic syndrome. **Results** The prevalence of MHO was 16.09% in the whole population investigated and 59.15% in individuals with obesity. The prevalence of MHO was significantly decreased with age in women ($P < 0.01$), but not significantly in men ($P > 0.05$). This proportion in rural residents was significantly higher than that in urban areas (64.75% vs.43.27%, $P < 0.01$). The Han nationality (OR = 0.33, 95%CI: 0.23 – 0.45), elevated waist circumference (WC, per 5 cm) (OR = 0.80, 95%CI: 0.73 – 0.88) and increased visceral fat index (VFI) level (OR = 0.80, 95%CI: 0.73 – 0.88) were significantly associated with a decreased risk of metabolically healthy phenotype in obese individuals. Moderate level of occupational physical activity (OR = 2.92, 95%CI: 1.75 – 4.88) was significantly associated with increased MHO risk. **Conclusions** The prevalence of MHO in Xinjiang population aged 35 – 80 years is high, especially in young people. Ethnicities, moderate level of occupational physical activity, WC, and VFI are the determinants associated with metabolic status in obesity.

Key words Metabolism; Obesity; Prevalence; Risk factors; Xinjiang area

肥胖是高血压、2 型糖尿病、血脂异常等心血管疾病的重要危险因素，同时与慢性疾病死亡率增高相关[1，2]。然而，并非所有肥胖患者的代谢疾病风险均增加。某些肥胖人群并未伴有血压、血糖升高、血脂异常等代谢异常，这类肥胖称为“代谢健康型肥胖”（metabolically healthy obese，MHO）[3，4]。研究显示，MHO 人群的心血管死亡率和全死因死亡率均低于代谢异常型肥胖（metabolically abnormal obese，MAO）患者[5，6]。美国人群 MHO 患病率为 9.70%，占肥胖人群的 31.70%[7]。中国人群 MHO 患病率为 3.91%，占肥胖人群 27.90%[8]。新疆地区居民肥胖及腹型肥胖患病率较高[9]。然而，关于 MHO 流行病学的调查研究较少，目前尚未有大规模具有代表性的抽样调查研究报道新疆地区 MHO 患病情况。本文旨在分析新疆地区 35 ~ 80 岁人群 MHO 患病情况及影响因素。

1. 对象与方法

1.1 对象

本研究调查对象来自于 2014 年公益性行业专项“西藏与新疆地区慢性心肺疾病现状调查研究”。此次调查采用分层多阶段随机抽样。首先在新疆维吾尔自治区内按城乡分为 2 层，在每层内采用与容量大小成比例的概率（probability proportional to size，PPS）抽取所需数量的区 / 县；然后在每个被抽中的区 / 县中采用简单随机抽样（simple random sampling，

SRS）方法抽取2个街道/乡镇；再在每个被抽中的街道/乡镇中采用SRS法抽取3个居委会/村委会；最后在被抽中的居委会/村委会中分性别、年龄采用SRS方法随机抽取调查15岁及以上个体，并对35岁及以上个体采集空腹血标本。共抽取新疆7个区县，2个城市地区，5个农村地区。本研究实际入选35～80岁调查对象4 627人，对完整且有效数据3 456（74.69%）人进行分析。本项研究通过中国医学科学院阜外医院伦理委员会批准，所有参与对象均签署知情同意书。

1.2 方法

采用横断面调查方法收集资料。调查内容包括问卷调查、体格检查和实验室检查。调查问卷内容包括：①基本信息：年龄、性别、婚姻状况、教育程度、行为习惯（吸烟、饮酒等）；②疾病史：如高血压、糖尿病、血脂异常等。体格检查：①血压：本次血压测量主要采用电子血压计（欧姆龙HBP-1300），要求调查对象在测量前30分钟内禁止剧烈活动或饮茶咖啡等兴奋性饮料，选择测量右上臂血压，测量前静坐5分钟。需连续测量3次，每两次间隔30秒，取3次的平均值作为个体血压值；②体重、体脂：采用体重体脂测量仪（欧姆龙V-BODY HBF-371）测量。体重体脂测量仪采用生物电阻抗法（bioelectrical impedance analysis，BIA）测量和计算身体脂肪率（body fat proportion，BFP）和内脏脂肪指数（visceral fat index，VFI），研究表明此类仪器可以准确地测量BFP和VFI[10]；③身高、腰围：采用标准身高计测量身高，统一的腰围尺测量腰围（waist circumference，WC）。按照身高和体重计算体重指数（body mass index，BMI），BMI = 体重（kg）/ 身高（m^2）。实验室标本：采集空腹12小时血标本，测量空腹血糖（fasting plasma glucose，FPG）、总胆固醇（total cholesterol，TC）、甘油三酯（triglyceride，TG）、高密度脂蛋白胆固醇（high density lipoprotein cholesterol，HDL-C）等生化指标。所有标本先保存于－70℃冰箱，由统一的实验室进行化验检测。所有生化检查采用美国贝克曼库尔特有限公司（Beckman Coulter, Inc.）AU400自动生化分析仪，试剂也为该公司制作。血糖采用葡萄糖氧化酶－过氧化物偶联体系（GOP-POD）方法测定，血脂采用酶法测定。

1.3 诊断标准

参照《中国成人超重和肥胖症预防控制指南》对不同BMI分类和定义：正常体重（BMI 18.5～23.9 kg/m^2）、超重（BMI 24.0～27.9 kg/m^2）、肥胖（BMI ≥ 28.0 kg/m^2）。参照《中国血脂异常指南》将男性腰围≥ 90 cm，女性腰围≥ 85 cm界定为中心性肥胖。代谢异常组分包括：①血压升高：收缩压≥ 130 mmHg或舒张压≥ 85 mmHg，或服用降压药物；②血糖水平升高：FPG ≥ 5.6 mmol/L，或服用降糖药物；③甘油三酯水平升高：TG ≥ 1.70 mmol/L；④高密度脂蛋白胆固醇（HDL-C）水平降低：< 1.04 mmol/L；⑤MHO定义为肥胖（BMI ≥ 28.0 kg/m^2）合并上述代谢异常组分数量≤ 1，MAO定义为肥胖合并代谢异常组分数量≥ 2。

吸烟定义为平均每日吸烟1支及以上，连续吸1年以上。饮酒定义为最近1个月每周至少饮酒 1 次。

1.4 质量控制

采用统一的调查方案、手册及问卷。所有相关工作人员均通过集中培训和考核，考核合格后方可参加调查。数据由项目组统一核查、整理。

1.5 统计学处理

采用 SAS 9.3 版进行数据整理和统计分析。计量资料使用（$\bar{x}$ ± SD）表示，两组比较采用 t 检验，多组比较采用 ANOVA 检验，两两比较采用 Bonferroni 法；计数资料用例数（%）表示，采用 χ^2 检验比较，率的趋势比较采用 Cochran-Armitage 趋势检验。多因素分析采用非条件 Logistic 回归。$P < 0.05$ 为差异有统计学意义。

2. 结果

2.1 调查对象的一般资料

本研究一共纳入新疆地区 35 ~ 80 岁人群 3 456 人，男性 1 659 人，占 48.00%。肥胖患病率为 27.20%，中心性肥胖率为 57.03%。该人群中 MHO 患病率为 16.09%，男性 229 例，占 13.80%，女性 327 例，占 18.20%，见表 1。

表 1 研究人群基线特征分布

项　目	男（n = 1 659）	女（n = 1 797）	合计（n = 3 456）
年龄（岁）	53.19 ± 12.52	53.80 ± 12.18	53.51 ± 12.35
汉族 [例（%）]	905（54.55）	850（47.30）**	1 755（50.78）
初中及以上 [例（%）]	840（50.63）	715（39.79）**	1 555（44.99）
职业劳动强度 [例（%）]			
无	321（19.35）	453（25.21）**	774（22.40）
轻	140（8.44）	90（5.01）	230（6.66）
中	312（18.81）	248（13.80）	560（16.20）
重	886（53.41）	1 006（55.98）	1 892（54.75）
吸烟 [例（%）]	751（45.27）	88（4.90）**	839（24.28）
饮酒 [例（%）]	274（16.52）	16（0.89）**	290（8.39）
中心性肥胖 [例（%）]	916（55.21）	1 055（58.71）*	1 971（57.03）

续表

项　　目	男（n＝1 659）	女（n＝1 797）	合计（n＝3 456）
TG（mmol/L）	1.39 ± 1.03	1.16 ± 0.72**	1.27 ± 0.89
HDL-C（mmol/L）	1.30 ± 0.29	1.44 ± 0.29**	1.37 ± 0.31
TC（mmol/L）	4.63 ± 0.86	4.69 ± 0.95*	4.66 ± 0.91
LDL-C（mmol/L）	2.73 ± 0.71	2.73 ± 0.77	2.73 ± 0.74
FPG（mmol/L）	5.48 ± 1.55	5.32 ± 1.3**	5.41 ± 1.43
SBP（mmHg）	129.52 ± 18.66	129.60 ± 21.26	129.56 ± 20.05
DBP（mmHg）	78.86 ± 11.25	75.54 ± 10.87**	77.15 ± 11.18
BMI（kg/m^2）	25.89 ± 3.52	26.14 ± 3.98*	26.02 ± 3.76
WC（cm）	90.81 ± 10.26	87.48 ± 10.91**	89.08 ± 10.73
BFP（%）	26.28 ± 5.16	34.97 ± 4.99**	30.80 ± 6.67
VFI	12.82 ± 4.97	9.34 ± 4.81**	11.01 ± 5.18
MHO[例（%）]	229（13.80）	327（18.20）**	556（16.09）

注：两组比较 * $P<0.05$，**$P<0.01$。

2.2　肥胖者中不同年龄段、性别、城乡的 MHO 患病率

肥胖人群中 MHO 患病率为 59.15%。女性 MHO 患病率显著高于男性（64.62% vs. 52.76%，$P<0.05$）。女性中 MHO 患病率随着年龄增加而下降（$P<0.01$），而男性未见该趋势（$P>0.05$）。农村居民 MHO 患病率显著高于城市（64.75% vs.43.27%，$P<0.01$）。城市居民中男女性肥胖患者中 MHO 患病率无统计学意义（$P>0.05$），见表 2。

表 2　不同年龄和性别肥胖人群中 MHO 和 MAO 患病率 [例（%）]

	男性		女性		合计	
	MHO	MAO	MHO	MAO	MHO	MAO
合计	229（52.76）	205（47.24）	327（64.62）*	179（35.38）	556（59.15）	384（40.85）
年龄段						
35 岁～	81（60.45）	53（39.55）	87（79.09）*	23（20.91）	168（68.85）	76（31.15）
45 岁～	66（48.53）	70（51.47）	108（68.79）*	49（31.21）	174（59.39）	119（40.61）
55 岁～	40（48.19）	43（51.81）	77（61.60）	48（38.40）	117（56.25）	91（43.75）

续表

	男性		女性		合计	
	MHO	MAO	MHO	MAO	MHO	MAO
65 岁 ~	32（55.17）	26（44.83）	42（55.26）	34（44.74）	74（55.22）	60（44.78）
75 ~ 80 岁	10（43.48）	13（56.52）	13（34.21）	25（66.79）	23（37.70）	38（62.30）
P for trend	> 0.05		< 0.01		< 0.01	
地区						
城市	52（40.31）△	77（59.69）	54（46.55）	62（53.45）	106（43.27）△	139（56.73）
农村	177（58.03）	128（41.97）	273（70.00）*	117（30.00）	450（64.75）	245（35.25）

注：与男性组比较 *$P < 0.01$；与农村组比较△ $P < 0.01$。

2.3 MHO 影响因素分析

先对自变量性别、年龄、民族、吸烟、饮酒、职业劳动强度、肥胖相关疾病家族史等进行单因素分析，见表 3。结果表明，与 MAO 患者相比，MHO 患者在自变量年龄、性别、民族、吸烟、饮酒、职业劳动强度差异有统计学意义（$P < 0.05$）。以是否患有 MHO 为因变量，以年龄、性别、民族、吸烟、饮酒、职业劳动强度为自变量进行多因素 Logistic 回归分析，结果表明，年龄增加、汉族（OR = 0.41，95%CI：0.30 ~ 0.56）、吸烟（OR = 0.63，95%CI：0.43 ~ 0.91）与 MHO 患病风险下降相关，中度职业体力劳动（OR = 2.63，95%CI：1.57 ~ 4.41）与 MHO 患病风险增加相关。纳入腰围（每 5 cm）模型中，腰围每增加 5 cm，MHO 患病风险下降 20%（OR = 0.80，95%CI：0.72 ~ 0.88），此时吸烟与 MHO 无关联；纳入 VFI 模型中，VFI 每升高一个等级（按三分位数将 VFI 分为低中高 3 个等级），MHO 患病风险下降 22%（OR = 0.78，95%CI：0.64 ~ 0.95）；而纳入 BFP 模型中并未发现 BFP 与 MHO 的显著关联。

表 3　MHO 影响因素的单因素和多因素 Logistic 回归分析

特征	OR（95%CI）				
	单因素	多因素	多因素 + WC	多因素 + VFI	多因素 + BFP
年龄段					
35 岁 ~	1.00（Reference）	1.00（Reference）	1.00（Reference）	1.00（Reference）	1.00（Reference）
45 岁 ~	0.66（0.46 ~ 0.95）	0.66（0.46 ~ 0.95）	0.58（0.39 ~ 0.86）	0.62（0.42 ~ 0.91）	0.57（0.40 ~ 0.84）
55 岁 ~	0.58（0.40 ~ 0.86）	0.58（0.40 ~ 0.86）	0.57（0.37 ~ 0.88）	0.60（0.39 ~ 0.93）	0.53（0.34 ~ 0.82）

续表

特 征	OR（95%CI）				
	单因素	多因素	多因素 + WC	多因素 + VFI	多因素 + BFP
65 岁 -	0.56（0.36 ~ 0.86）	0.56（0.36 ~ 0.86）	0.62（0.37 ~ 1.00）	0.63（0.38 ~ 1.04）	0.52（0.31 ~ 0.88）
75 ~ 80 岁	0.27（0.15 ~ 0.49）	0.27（0.15 ~ 0.49）	0.34（0.18 ~ 0.66）	0.35（0.17 ~ 0.67）	0.29（0.15 ~ 0.57）
性别					
男	1.00（Reference）	1.00（Reference）	1.00（Reference）	1.00（Reference）	1.00（Reference）
女	1.64（1.26 ~ 2.13）	1.34（0.98 ~ 1.85）	1.20（0.87 ~ 1.66）	1.09（0.76 ~ 1.55）	1.62（1.01 ~ 2.61）
民族					
其他民族	1.00（Reference）	1.00（Reference）	1.00（Reference）	1.00（Reference）	1.00（Reference）
汉族	0.44（0.34 ~ 0.57）	0.41（0.30 ~ 0.56）	0.34（0.25 ~ 0.47）	0.38（0.28 ~ 0.52）	0.40（0.29 ~ 0.54）
吸烟					
否	1.00（Reference）	1.00（Reference）	1.00（Reference）	1.00（Reference）	1.00（Reference）
是	0.61（0.44 ~ 0.84）	0.63（0.43 ~ 0.91）	0.68（0.47 ~ 1.00）	0.63（0.43 ~ 0.91）	0.63（0.43 ~ 0.92）
饮酒					
否	1.00（Reference）	1.00（Reference）	1.00（Reference）	1.00（Reference）	1.00（Reference）
是	0.58（0.35 ~ 0.99）	0.93（0.53 ~ 1.64）	0.97（0.55 ~ 1.73）	0.93（0.52 ~ 1.63）	0.92（0.52 ~ 1.62）
职业劳动强度					
无	1.00（Reference）	1.00（Reference）	1.00（Reference）	1.00（Reference）	1.00（Reference）
轻	0.56（0.30 ~ 1.06）	0.56（0.28 ~ 1.14）	0.61（0.30 ~ 1.23）	0.59（0.30 ~ 1.20）	0.57（0.28 ~ 1.14）
中	1.99（1.29 ~ 3.08）	2.63（1.57 ~ 4.41）	2.70（1.60 ~ 4.57）	2.72（1.62 ~ 4.59）	2.66（1.58 ~ 4.48）
重	1.58（1.13 ~ 2.22）	1.36（0.94 ~ 1.98）	1.40（0.96 ~ 2.05）	1.40（0.96 ~ 2.04）	1.38（0.95 ~ 2.01）
疾病家族史	0.85（0.657 ~ 1.11）	0.78（0.59 ~ 1.03）	0.80（0.60 ~ 1.06） 0.79（0.60 ~ 1.05）	0.78（0.59 ~ 1.03）	
WC/VFI /BFP	~	~	0.80（0.72 ~ 0.88）	0.78（0.64 ~ 0.95）	0.86（0.65 ~ 1.14）

注：WC：腰围（每 5 cm）；VFI：内脏脂肪指数（按三分位数分组，低：1 ~ 15，中：16 ~ 18，高：19 ~ 30）；BFP：身体脂肪率（按三分位数分组，低：5.0% ~ 31.9%，中：32.0% ~ 38.6%，高：38.7% ~ 50.0%）。

3. 讨论

本研究显示新疆地区 35 ~ 80 岁居民肥胖患病率为 27.20%，MHO 患病率为 16.09%，肥胖人群中 MHO 患病率为 59.15%，MAO 患病率为 40.85%。说明新疆地区肥胖较为严重，半数以上肥胖人群表现代谢健康状态。肥胖人群中，年龄增加、汉族、WC 增加、VFI 升高以及吸烟与 MHO 患病风险下降相关，中度职业体力劳动与 MHO 风险增加相关，即年龄增加、汉族、WC 增加、VFI 升高与肥胖人群中代谢异常状态有关。高脂肪、高碳水化合物饮食，蔬菜水果摄入较少，可能是新疆地区肥胖问题较为严重的主要原因。

由于研究对象特征不同，以及代谢健康和肥胖的定义不一致，现有研究报道的 MHO 患病率范围不等。本研究显示，新疆居民 MHO 患病率为 16.09%，肥胖人群中超过 1 /2 表现为 MHO，高于大部分欧美研究。Wildman 等[7] 报道 20 岁以上美国人群和肥胖患者 MHO 患病率分别为 9.70% 和 31.70%。瑞典一项对 35 ~ 75 岁人群的研究显示，根据不同 MHO 定义，男性 MHO 患病率范围为 3.30 ~ 32.10%，女性为 11.40 ~ 43.30%，其中最接近本研究的定义估计的 MHO 患病率为男性 39.00%，女性 30.10%[11]。我国 35 ~ 72 岁普通人群和肥胖人群中 MHO 患病率分别为 3.91% 和 27.90%[12]，低于新疆地区。其样本未包含新疆居民，研究对象主要来自我国东部地区可能与其 MHO 患病率低于本研究有关。新疆地区 MHO 患病率也高于其他亚洲人群，如日本和印度，其普通人群和肥胖人群中 MHO 患病率分别为 8.89% 和 44.06%[13]，13.30% 和 47.33%[8]。造成新疆地区 MHO 患病率较高的原因可能是新疆为多民族聚居地区，且由于气候环境等原因，当地居民生活饮食习惯较独特。

无论采用何种 MHO 定义，多数研究均显示男性和女性 MHO 患病率随着年龄增加而下降[4]。本研究肥胖女性 MHO 患病率随着年龄上升呈下降趋势，男性未观察到该趋势。年轻男性 MHO 患病率较女性低，35 ~ 44、45 ~ 54 岁年龄段中肥胖男性健康代谢型患病率低于肥胖女性，而 55 ~ 80 岁人群中患病率无性别差异。该结果可能与体重、体成分中脂肪含量随着年龄上升而增加，女性激素水平随着年龄增加而下降，尤其绝经后雌激素水平下降、腹部脂肪堆积[14] 有关。本研究还发现新疆农村地区 MHO 比例高于城市，农村居民 MHO 患病率存在性别差异，而城市居民无差异。可能与城市地区膳食脂肪和酒精等摄入量高于农村，且农村居民职业性体力劳动强度较大有关。

本研究显示，部分人口学特征和行为方式与 MHO 有关。适度体力活动可减轻但并不能消除肥胖对心血管健康的不利影响[15, 16]。大量研究显示，适度体力活动与 MHO 呈正相关[11, 17, 18]。本研究结果与之一致。汉族 MHO 患病风险比其他民族（主要为哈萨克族、蒙古族、回族和维吾尔族）低 67.00%。汉族和少数民族生活方式及遗传因素等差异可能是汉族 MHO 患病率较低的原因之一。WC 增加与 MAO 患病风险增加相关，与大部分研究结果相同[7, 12]。然而有研究显示 WC 增加与 MHO 患病风险降低并无显著关联[17]。WC 增加可能是腹部皮下脂肪或者内脏脂肪或两者均增加导致[19]，仅通过 WC 并不能分辨皮下脂肪和内脏脂肪对 MHO 的影响。本研究中调整 VFI 模型结果显示，VFI 增加与 MHO 风险下降有关。提示内脏脂肪含量增加与肥胖患者代谢异常风险增加有关。本研究中调整 BFP 的模型中未观察到 BFP 与 MHO 的关联，可能与肥胖人群 BFP 均较高有关。提示肥胖人群中控制腰围的同时不能忽视对内脏脂肪含量的关注。

本研究基于大规模且具有代表性的抽样调查，但也存在一定局限性。首先，尽管研究对象具有代表性，但对 MHO 患病率的民族差异还需要进一步研究；第二，研究缺乏饮食相关资料；第三，研究为横断面调查，对因果推断具有局限性，因此 MHO 与其影响因素的深层关系需要前瞻性研究进一步证实。

MHO 的心血管事件风险虽然低于 MAO，但仍较高，提示 MHO 并不是一个健康状态 [20]。新疆地区 MHO 患病率较高，提示在制定有效的防控策略控制肥胖同时，应积极监测相关代谢指标及其变化，如血压、血糖和血脂，以期降低总体心血管疾病风险。其次，解决肥胖问题时不能“一刀切”，需结合体型和代谢类型对肥胖进行分层，针对性制定治疗和干预措施更有利于肥胖及相关代谢性疾病的防控。

参考文献

[1] Mokdad AH, Ford ES, Bowman BA, et al. Prevalence of obesity, diabetes, and obesity-related health risk factors, 2001[J]. Jama, 2003, 289(1): 76-79.

[2] Van Gaal LF, Mertens IL, De Block CE. Mechanisms linking obesity with cardiovascular disease[J]. Nature, 2006, 444(7121): 875-880.

[3] Rey-Lopez JP, de Rezende LF, Pastor-Valero M, et al. The prevalence of metabolically healthy obesity: a systematic review and critical evaluation of the definitions used[J]. Obes Rev, 2014, 15(10): 781-790.

[4] Phillips CM. Metabolically healthy obesity: definitions, determinants and clinical implications[J]. Rev Endocr Metab Disord, 2013, 14(3): 219-227.

[5] Kramer CK, Zinman B, Retnakaran R. Are metabolically healthy overweight and obesity benign conditions: A systematic review and meta-analysis[J]. Ann Intern Med, 2013, 159(11): 758-769.

[6] Hamer M, Stamatakis E. Metabolically healthy obesity and risk of allcause and cardiovascular disease mortality[J]. J Clin Endocrinol Metab, 2012, 97(7): 2482-2488.

[7] Wildman RP, Muntner P, Reynolds K, et al. The obese without cardiometabolic risk factor clustering and the normal weight with cardiometabolic risk factor clustering: prevalence and correlates of 2 phenotypes among the US population (NHANES 1999-2004) [J]. Arch Intern Med, 2008, 168(15): 1617-1624.

[8] Geetha L, Deepa M, Anjana RM, et al. Prevalence and clinical profile of metabolic obesity and phenotypic obesity in Asian Indians [J]. J Diabetes Sci Technol, 2011, 5(2): 439-446.

[9] 何佳，郭恒，丁玉松，等. 新疆哈萨克族、维吾尔族和汉族农村居民超重、肥胖流行病学调查 [J]. 中华流行病学杂志，2013, 34(12): 1164-1168.

[10] Bosy-Westphal A, Later W, Hitze B, et al. Accuracy of bioelectrical impedance consumer devices for measurement of body composition in comparison to whole body magnetic resonance imaging and dual X-ray absorpti-

ometry [J]. Obes Facts, 2008, 1(6): 319-324.

[11] Velho S, Paccaud F, Waeber G, et al. Metabolically healthy obesity: different prevalences using different criteria [J]. Eur J Clin Nutr, 2010, 64(10): 1043-1051.

[12] Zheng R, Yang M, Bao Y, et al. Prevalence and Determinants of Metabolic Health in Subjects with Obesity in Chinese Population [J]. Int J Environ Res Public Health, 2015, 12(11): 13662-13677.

[13] Heianza Y, Arase Y, Tsuji H, et al. Metabolically healthy obesity, presence or absence of fatty liver, and risk of type 2 diabetes in Japanese individuals: Toranomon Hospital Health Management Center Study 20 (TOPICS 20) [J]. J Clin Endocrinol Metab, 2014, 99(8): 2952-2960.

[14] Otsuki M, Kasayama S, Morita S, et al. Menopause, but not age, is an independent risk factor for fasting plasma glucose levels in nondiabetic women[J]. Menopause, 2007, 14(3 Pt 1): 404-407.

[15] Hu G, Tuomilehto J, Silventoinen K, et al. Joint effects of physical activity, body mass index, waist circumference and waist-to-hip ratio with the risk of cardiovascular disease among middle-aged Finnish men and women[J]. Eur Heart J, 2004, 25(24): 2212-2219.

[16] Li TY, Rana JS, Manson JE, et al. Obesity as compared with physical activity in predicting risk of coronary heart disease in women[J]. Circulation, 2006, 113(4): 499-506.

[17] Lopez-Garcia E, Guallar-Castillon P, Leon-Munoz L, et al. Prevalence and determinants of metabolically healthy obesity in Spain[J]. Atherosclerosis, 2013, 231(1): 152-157.

[18] Aparicio VA, Soriano-Maldonado A, Buitrago F, et al. The Role of Sex and Domestic Physical Activity on the Metabolically Healthy and Unhealthy Obesity. The HERMEX Study [J]. Rev Esp Cardiol (Engl Ed), 2016, 69(10): 983-986.

[19] Preis SR, Massaro JM, Robins SJ, et al. Abdominal subcutaneous and visceral adipose tissue and insulin resistance in the Framingham heart study [J]. Obesity (Silver Spring), 2010, 18 (11): 2191-2198.

[20] Fan J, Song Y, Chen Y, et al. Combined effect of obesity and cardiometabolic abnormality on the risk of cardiovascular disease: a meta analysis of prospective cohort study [J]. Int J Cardiol, 2013, 168(5): 4761-4768.

新疆、西藏地区35岁及以上人群身体脂肪率、内脏脂肪指数与心脏代谢性危险因素聚集的关系△

王佳丽，陈　祚，张林峰，王　馨，董　莹，聂静雨，郑聪毅，邵　澜，田　野，王增武

中国医学科学院阜外医院，国家心血管病中心社区防治部　北京.102308

通讯作者：王增武，E-mail：wangzengwu@foxmail.com

摘　要　目的　探讨我国新疆、西藏地区35岁及以上人群身体脂肪率（BFP）和内脏脂肪指数（VFI）与心脏代谢性危险因素聚集的关系。**方法**　2015～2016年，采用分层多阶段随机抽样，选取新疆、西藏地区35岁及以上调查对象7 571人，有效数据5 643人。危险因素聚集定义为两种及以上危险因素（高血压、糖尿病、高甘油三酯血症、低高密度脂蛋白胆固醇血症）同时存在。采用Logistic回归和受试者工作特征（ROC）曲线进行分析。**结果**　新疆、西藏地区35岁及以上居民危险因素聚集患病率为9.78%。BFP、VFI按照四分位数分组，调整性别、年龄、民族、吸烟、饮酒、教育程度、职业劳动强度和海拔后，随着BFP或VFI水平升高，BFP或VFI与危险因素聚集关联的OR值增大。以BFP为5.0%～27.0%组OR值为1，BFP为27.1%～31.7%组、31.8%～36.6%组和36.7%～50.0%组OR值（95%CI）分别为1.15（0.86～1.54）、1.48（1.05～2.07）和1.72（1.10～2.68）；以VFI为1～6组OR值为1，VFI为7～9组、10～13组和14～30组OR值（95%CI）分别为1.20（0.81～1.79）、1.91（1.30～2.80）和3.91（2.64～5.77）。BFP、VFI预测危险因素聚集的曲线下面积（AUC）分别为0.55和0.70，差异有统计学意义（$P < 0.01$）。**结论**　BFP和VFI水平与心脏代谢性危险因素聚集相关，VFI对危险因素聚集的预测价值较好。

关键词　身体脂肪率；内脏脂肪指数；心脏代谢性危险因素聚集

△　本文发表于：中华流行病学杂志，2017，38（6）：727-731.

Association between Body Fat Percentage, Visceral Fat Index and Cardiometabolic Risk Factor Clustering among Population Aged 35 Year Old or Over in Tibet Autonomous Region and Xinjiang Uygur Autonomous Region

Wang Iiali, Chen Zuo, Zhang Linfeng, Wang Xin, Dong Ying, Nie Jingyu, Zheng Congyi, Shao Lan, Tian Ye, Wang Zengwu, for the Croup of Study on Prevalence of Chronic Cardiopulmonary Disease in Tibet and Xinjiang Area

Division of Prevention and Community Health, National Center for Cardiovascular Diseases; Fuwai Hospital, PUMC and CAMS, Beijing 102308, China

Corresponding author: Wang Zengwu, Email: wangzengwu@foxmail. com

Abstract **Objective** To investigate the association between body fat percentage (BFP), visceral fat index (VFI), and cardiometabolic risk factor clustering (CRFC) among population aged 35 or older in Tibet and Xinjiang regions. **Methods** Using the stratified multi-stage random sampling method, we investigated 7 571 residents aged 35 or above with international standardized examination between 2015 and 2016. Of the eligible 5 643 participants, association of BFP and VFI with CRFC was defined as having two or more of the four risk factors hypertension, diabetes mellitus, high TG and low HDL-C at the same time. Logistic regression analysis and receiver operating characteristic (ROC) curve analysis were employed to further explore the relationships. **Results** The overall prevalence of CRFC among aged 35 and older population in Tibet and Xinjiang regions was 9.78%. BFP and VFI were divided into four groups by quartile. After adjustment for age, gender, race, cigarette smoking, alcohol consumption, education attainments, and altitude of residence, ORs of CRFC seemed to have increased with BFP and VFI. Compared with people having BFP of 5.0% - 27.0%, the OR (95%CI) were 1.15 (0.86 - 1.54), 1.48 (1.05 - 2.07) and 1.72 (1.10 - 2.68) for the ones who presented 27. 1% - 31.7%, 31.8% - 36.6% and 36.7% - 50.0% of BFP. Compared to people of having 1 - 6 of VFI, with OR (95%CI) as 1.20 (0.81 - 1.79), 1.91 (1.30 - 2.80) and 3.91 (2.64 - 5.77) for the ones having 7 - 9, 10 - 13 and 14 - 30 of VFI. Areas under the curve (AUC) of CRFC appeared as 0.55 for BFP and 0.70 for VFI, respectively, with statistically significant difference ($P < 0.01$). **Conclusions** Both BFP and VFI levels are closely associated with CRFC while VFI may have a better predictive value than the BFP.

Key words Body fat percentage; Visceral fat index; Cardiometabolic risk factors clustering

肥胖与心血管疾病危险因素及其聚集密切相关，尤其是中心性肥胖 [1-2]。我国人群超重、肥胖患病率呈持续上升趋势 [3]。肥胖相关慢性疾病的发病率和死亡率亦显著增加。肥胖已成为重要公共卫生问题。目前普遍采用 BMI 和腰围（WC）作为评价肥胖及内脏脂肪蓄积的指标。有研究提示身体脂肪率（body fat percentage，BFP）和内脏脂肪指数（visceral fat index，VFI）对心脏代谢性危险因素的预测效果可能更优[4-9]，但目前尚无定论[10]。在我国人群中，尤其是新疆、西藏，BFP 和 VFI 的应用价值尚缺乏充分证据。本研究利用新疆、西藏项目调查人群的数据进行分析，探讨 BFP 和 VFI 与心脏代谢性危险因素聚集的关系及其预测价值。

1. 对象与方法

1.1　研究对象

本研究采用分层多阶段随机抽样。首先分别在西藏自治区和新疆维吾尔自治区内按城乡分为 2 层，在每层内采用与容量大小成比例的概率（PPS）抽取所需数量的区 / 县；然后在被抽中的区 / 县中采用简单随机抽样（SRS）方法抽取 2 个街道 / 乡镇；再在被抽中的街道 / 乡镇中采用 SRS 法抽取 3 个居委会 / 村委会；最后在被抽中的居委会 / 村委会中分性别、年龄采用 SRS 方法随机抽取调查≥ 15 岁个体，并对≥ 35 岁个体采集空腹血标本。抽取新疆 7 个地区，西藏 6 个地区。本研究实际入选≥ 35 岁调查对象 7 571 人，对数据完整的 5 643 人进行分析。本项研究通过中国医学科学院阜外医院伦理委员会批准，所有参加对象均签署知情同意书。

1.2　研究方法

采用横断面调查方法收集资料。内容包括问卷调查、体格检查和实验室检查。

（1）调查问卷内容包括：①基本信息：年龄、性别、婚姻状况、文化程度、行为习惯（吸烟、饮酒等）；②疾病史：如脑卒中、糖尿病、血脂异常等。

（2）体格检查：①血压：采用电子血压计（欧姆龙 HBP-1300），要求调查对象在测量前 30 min 禁止剧烈活动或饮茶咖啡等兴奋性饮料，选择测量右上臂的血压，测量前静坐 5 min。需连续测量 3 次，每两次间隔 30 s，取平均值作为个体的血压值；②体重、BFP 和 VFI：采用生物电阻抗法体重体脂测量仪（欧姆龙 V-BODY HBF-371）测量，此类仪器可以准确地测量 PBF 和 VFI[11]。

（3）实验室标本：采集空腹 12 h 血标本，测量 FPG、TC、TG、HDL-C 等生化指标。所有标本先保存于－70℃冰箱，由统一的实验室进行化验检测。所有生化检查采用美国贝克曼库尔特有限公司（Beckman Coulter，Inc.）AU400 自动生化分析仪和试剂。血糖采用葡萄糖氧化酶－过氧化物偶联体系（GOP-POD）方法测定，血脂采用酶法测定。

1.3 诊断标准

①高血压诊断标准采用2010年中国高血压防治指南推荐的标准：SBP ≥ 140 mmHg（1mmHg = 0.133 kPa）或 DBP ≥ 90 mmHg，对既往确诊的高血压患者或在两周内服用过降压药者，不论检查时血压是否异常均诊断为高血压；②糖尿病定义为既往确诊或实验室检查 FPG ≥ 7.0 mmol/L；③血脂异常采用 2007 年中国成人血脂异常指南推荐的标准：高甘油三酯血症定义为 TG ≥ 2.26 mmol/L，低高密度脂蛋白胆固醇血症定义为 HDL-C < 1.04 mmol/L；④危险因素聚集指在上述 4 项危险因素中，同一个体同时具有 2 项及以上危险因素；⑤吸烟者定义为平均每日吸烟 1 支及以上，并连续吸 1 年以上；⑥饮酒定义为最近 1 个月每周至少饮酒 1 次。

1.4 质量控制

调查中采用统一的调查方案、手册及问卷。调查前，牵头单位负责组织各调查单位所有项目参与人员集中培训和考核。考核合格后方可参加调查。

1.5 统计学分析

采用 EpiData 3.1 软件建立数据库，SAS 9.3 及 MedCalc 17.0.4 软件进行统计学分析。计量资料使用 $\bar{x}$ ± SD 表示，计数资料用人数和构成比（%）描述。采用非条件 Logistic 回归模型分析 BFP、VFI 与危险因素聚集的关系。采用受试者工作特征（ROC）曲线比较 BFP 和 VFI 对危险因素聚集的预测价值。以 $P < 0.05$ 为差异有统计学意义。

2. 结果

2.1 基本情况

男性 2 560 人，占 45.36%。男性中 VFI 水平、汉族所占比例、吸烟率、饮酒率、职业劳动强度重的比例、初中及以上文化程度比例及危险因素聚集患病率均显著高于女性（$P < 0.01$）。见表 1。

表 1　新疆、西藏 35 岁及以上人群基线特征分布

特　征	男性（$n = 2\,560$）	女性（$n = 3\,083$）	合计（$n = 5\,643$）	P 值
年龄（岁，$\bar{x}$ ± SD）	53.3 ± 12.96	53.67 ± 12.28	53.51 ± 12.6	0.27
汉族	1 036（40.47）	949（30.78）	1 985（35.18）	< 0.01
吸烟	1 037（40.51）	122（3.96）	1 159（20.54）	< 0.01

续表

特　征	男性（n = 2 560）	女性（n = 3 083）	合计（n = 5 643）	P 值
饮酒	440（17.19）	96（3.11）	536（9.50）	< 0.01
初中及以上学历	1 067（41.68）	894（29.00）	1 961（34.75）	< 0.01
职业性劳动强度				< 0.01
无	677（26.45）	1 208（39.18）	1 885（33.40）	
轻	280（10.94）	164（5.32）	444（7.87）	
中	543（21.21）	481（15.60）	1 024（18.15）	
重	1 060（41.41）	1 230（39.90）	2 290（40.58）	
高血压	909（35.51）	1 119（36.30）	2 028（35.94）	0.54
高甘油三酯血症	259（10.12）	145（4.70）	404（7.16）	< 0.01
低高密度脂蛋白胆固醇血症	392（15.31）	164（5.32）	556（9.85）	< 0.01
糖尿病	191（7.46）	176（5.71）	367（6.50）	< 0.00
危险因素聚集	325（12.70）	227（7.36）	552（9.78）	< 0.01
身体脂肪率（%，$\bar{x}$ ± SD）	27.18 ± 5.67	35.46 ± 5.31	31.70 ± 6.85	< 0.01
内脏脂肪指数（$\bar{x}$ ± SD）	12.43 ± 5.17	9.33 ± 4.94	10.73 ± 5.28	< 0.01
海拔（m）				< 0.01
< 1 000	1 200（46.88）	1 269（41.16）	2 469（43.75）	
1 000 ~	802（31.33）	919（29.81）	1 721（30.50）	
> 3 500	558（21.80）	895（29.03）	1 453（25.75）	

注：括号外数据为人数，括号内数据为构成比（%）。吸烟定义为平均每日吸烟 1 支及以上，并连续吸 1 年以上；饮酒定义为最近 1 个月每周至少饮酒 1 次。

2.2 BFP、VFI 人群中危险因素及其聚集的分布情况

BFP 四分位不同组间，高血压、糖尿病、高甘油三酯血症、低高密度脂蛋白胆固醇血症和危险因素聚集率差异有统计学意义（P < 0.05）。两两比较显示，按 BFP 四分位分组，第一组和第二组、第一组和第四组以及第二组和第三组间差异有统计学意义（P < 0.008 3）。由 BFP 低到高四组的危险因素聚集患病率分别为 7.60%、10.81%、8.80% 和 10.97%。见图 1。

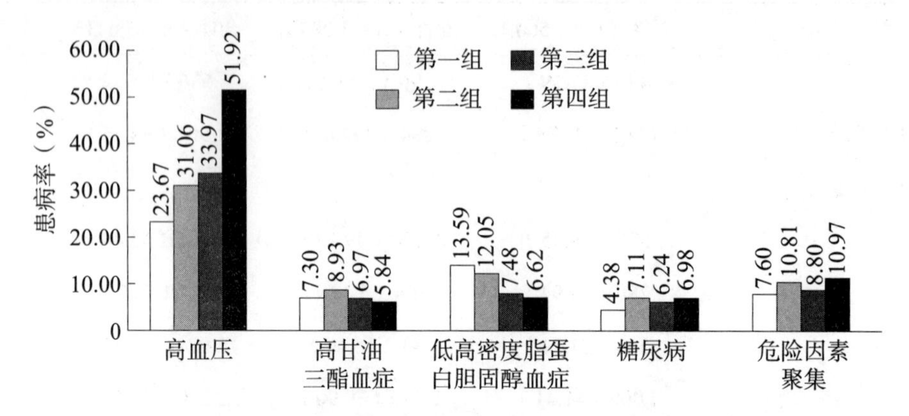

图 1　不同身体脂肪率分组中各项危险因素及其聚集的患病率

注：运用四分位数法将体脂脂肪分为：第一组 5.0% ~ 27.0%，第二组：27.1% ~ 31.7%，第三组 31.8% ~ 36.6%，第四组：36.70% ~ 50.0%。

VFI 四分位不同组间，高血压、糖尿病、高 TG 血症、低 HDL-C 血症和危险因素聚集率差异有统计学意义（$P < 0.05$）。两两比较显示，按 VFI 四分位分组，除第一组和第二组间无差异，其余各组间差异均有统计学意义（$P < 0.008\ 3$）。由 VFI 低到高四组的危险因素聚集患病率分别为 3.68%、5.11%、9.19% 和 18.60%。高血压、糖尿病、高 TG 血症、低 HDL-C 血症和危险因素聚集患病率均随着 VFI 升高呈上升趋势。见图 2。

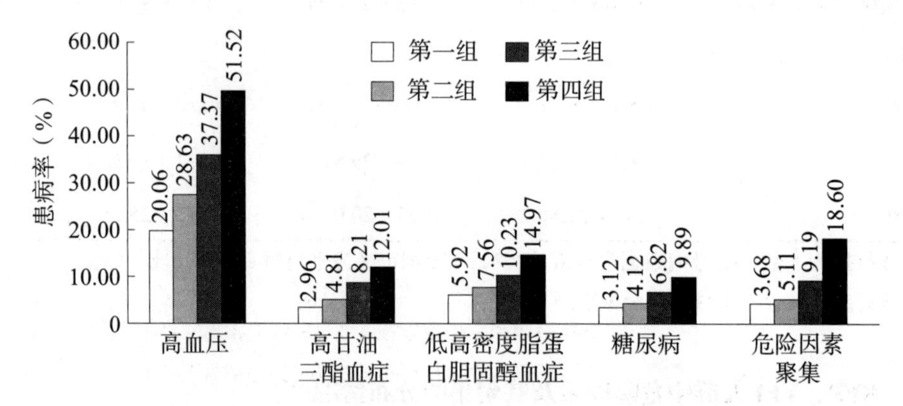

图 2　不同内脏脂肪指数分组中各项危险因素及其聚集的患病率

注：运用四分位数法将内脏脂肪指数分为：第一组：1 ~ 6，第二组：7 ~ 9，第三组：10 ~ 13，第四组：14 ~ 30。

2.3　多因素分析 BFP、VFI 与危险因素聚集

以危险因素聚集为因变量，采用多因素 Logistic 回归分析不同 BFP、VFI 水平对各项危险因素及其聚集的影响。BFP、VFI 按照四分位数分组，调整性别、年龄、民族、吸

烟、饮酒、教育程度、职业劳动强度和海拔，结果显示，随着BFP或VFI水平升高，BFP或VFI与危险因素聚集关联的OR值增大。以BFP为5.0%～27.0%组OR值为1，BFP为27.1%～31.7%组、31.8%～36.6%组和36.7%～50.0%组OR值（95%CI）分别为1.15（0.86～1.54）、1.48（1.05～2.07）和1.72（1.10～2.68）；以VFI为1～6组OR值为1，VFI为7～9组、10～13组和14～30组OR值（95%CI）分别为1.20（0.81～1.79）、1.91（1.30～2.80）和3.91（2.64～5.77）。BFP ≥ 31.6%和VFI ≥ 10是心脏代谢性危险因素聚集的独立危险因素。见表2。

表2　不同BFP、VFI水平对各项危险因素及其聚集的影响（标化OR值及95%CI）

特征		高血压标化 OR值（95%CI）	高TG血症 OR值（95%CI）	低HDL-C血症 OR值（95%CI）	糖尿病 OR值（95%CI）	危险因素聚集 OR值（95%CI）
BFP	Q1	1 00	1.00	1.00	1.00	1.00
	Q2	1.21（0.99～1.47）	1.28（0.93～1.76）	0.95（0.73～1.24）	1.46（1.02～2.11）	1.15（0.86～1.54）
	Q3	1.48（1.19～1.85）	1.86（1.27～2.72）	0.88（0.64～1.22）	1.57（1.03～2.39）	1.48（1.05～2.07）
	Q4	1.99（1.51～2.62）	1.93（1.14～3.25）	0.94（0.61～1.46）	1.48（0.86～2.56）	1.72（1.10～2.68）
VFI	Q1	1.00	1.00	1.00	1.00	1.00
	Q2	1.32（1.07～1.62）	1.41（0.91～2.17）	1.26（0.90～1.75）	1.24（0.80～1.93）	1.20（0.81～1.79）
	Q3	1.83（1.48～2.26）	2.15（1.41～3.29）	1.56（1.12～2.17）	1.87（1.21～2.89）	1.91（1.30～2.80）
	Q4	2.81（2.24～3.53）	3.12（1.99～4.89）	2.49（1.75～3.54）	2.48（1.57～3.93）	3.91（2.64～5.77）

注：调整性别、年龄、民族、吸烟、饮酒、教育程度、职业劳动强度和海拔。

2.4　BFP、VFI对各项危险因素及其聚集的预测价值

BFP、VFI预测危险因素聚集、糖尿病、高甘油三酯血症的ROC曲线下面积（95%CI）分别为0.55（0.53～0.56）和0.70（0.68～0.71）、0.55（0.54～0.57）和0.63（0.62～0.65）以及0.52（0.51～0.54）和0.65（0.64～0.66），VFI对危险因素聚集、糖尿病和高甘油三酯血症预测的ROC曲线下面积均大于BFP（$P<0.01$）。见表3。

表3　身体脂肪率和内脏脂肪指数对危险因素及其聚集的受试者工作特征分析

特征	身体脂肪率		内脏脂肪指数		AUC	95%CI	*P*值
	AUC	95%CI	AUC	95%CI			
危险因素聚集	0.55	0.53～0.56	0.70	0.68～0.71	0.14	0.11～0.17	<0.01
高血压	0.64	0.62～0.65	0.65	0.64～0.67	0.02	0.00～0.03	0 06

续表

特征	身体脂肪率		内脏脂肪指数		AUC	95%CI	*P* 值
	AUC	95%CI	AUC	95%CI			
糖尿病	0.55	0.54 ~ 0.57	0.63	0.62 ~ 0.65	0.08	0.05 ~ 0.11	< 0.01
高胆固醇血症	0.52	0.51 ~ 0.54	0.65	0.64 ~ 0.66	0.12	0.08 ~ 0.17	< 0.01
低高密度脂蛋白胆固醇血症	0.59	0.57 ~ 0.60	0.61	0.60 ~ 0.62	0.02	0.02 ~ 0.05	0 34

注：AUC 为曲线下面积。

3. 讨论

肥胖与心血管疾病危险因素及其聚集密切相关[12-13]，探索肥胖相关的有效筛查指标以预测心血管危险因素聚集在慢病防治中具有重要意义。本研究结果显示，BFP、VFI 水平均与心脏代谢性危险因素聚集相关，VFI 对危险因素聚集的预测价值较好。

我国新疆、西藏地区危险因素聚集患病率相对较高，男性 12.70%，女性 7.36%。其中男性高甘油三酯血症、低高密度脂蛋白胆固醇血症和糖尿病患病率均高于女性。国内一项研究显示，2 项以上危险因素聚集（高血压、糖尿病、血脂异常）患病率男性（37.0%）显著高于女性（14.4%）[7]，本研究与之一致。危险因素聚集患病率相对较高可能与新疆、西藏居民饮食多为肉类等高热量高脂低纤维食物以及气候寒冷及环境受限，人们缺少体育锻炼有关。既往研究报道，女性 BFP 更高[14]。本研究中女性 BFP 高于男性，但男性 VFI 显著高于女性。研究发现内脏型肥胖对心血管健康的影响更密切[15]，这可能是男性危险因素聚集患病率高的原因之一。男性吸烟、饮酒率高于女性，女性健康意识较强等可部分解释危险因素的性别差异，提示当地居民应适当控制摄入高热量食物，增加体育运动。

既往研究发现，高 BFP 水平可增加心血管疾病的发病风险，且该效应独立于 BMI 的影响[6]；VFI 与 MS 及其各成分也密切相关，MS 患病风险随 VFI 升高而增加[9,16]。亚洲人 BMI 水平较低，但在相同的 BMI 水平中，其 BFP 水平较高[17]。本调查发现，BFP、VFI 均与代谢性危险因素聚集相关，高血压、糖尿病、高甘油三酯血症、低高密度脂蛋白胆固醇血症和危险因素聚集患病率均随着 VFI 水平的升高而增加；调整混杂因素后，BFP 和 VFI 水平升高仍与代谢性危险因素聚集的患病风险呈正相关。

本研究利用 ROC 曲线分析，提示 BFP 和 VFI 对高血压均有一定预测价值，与一项对我国 35 ~ 64 岁人群的研究结果一致[18]。研究显示，VFI 对危险因素聚集的预测价值较高，且 VFI 对危险因素聚集、糖尿病、高甘油三酯血症的预测价值均优于 BFP。Knowles 等[19]的研究也发现 VFI 是 MS 及其组分较好的预测工具。国内一项研究也证明 VFI 在男女中均能较好预测 MS[20]。相比于身体脂肪，内脏脂肪与危险因素聚集关系更为密切[21]。腰围虽为间接评价内脏脂肪的指标，但其并不能区分皮下脂肪和内脏脂肪的质量[22]。VFI 比腰围能更加准确反映内脏脂肪含量[23]，区分内脏脂肪和皮下脂肪。提示脂肪堆积和/或内脏脂肪堆积可能是心血管代谢异常和其他危险因素聚集的重要预测因素。

本研究基于大规模且具有代表性的抽样调查，但也存在一定局限性。研究为横断面调查，BFP、VFI 与危险因素聚集的深层关系需要前瞻性研究进一步证实。本研究提示，VFI 与心脏代谢性危险因素聚集关系紧密，VFI 可作为一个简便筛查工具，对高血压、糖尿病、危险因素聚集等的高危人群筛查和家庭健康监测具有重要意义。对肥胖相关心血管代谢性疾病的预防，不仅要关注脂肪含量，脂肪分布亦不容忽视。高危人群应倡导健康生活方式，预防相关疾病的发生发展。

致谢

感谢参与项目的所有专家及所有调查人员；协作组组成单位及主要调查人员：国家心血管病中心中国医学科学院阜外医院：王增武、张林峰、陈祚、王馨、邵澜、郭敏、田野、赵天明、范围辉、董莹、聂静雨、王佳丽、郑聪毅、贾秀云、朱曼璐、王文、陈伟伟、高润霖；卫生部北京医院：郭岩斐、孙铁英、王玉霞、柴迪、马雅立、仝亚琪；中国人民解放军总医院：陈韵岱、冯斌、朱庆磊、周珊珊、刘杰、王晶、杨丽娜、杨瑛、段鹏；新疆维吾尔自治区人民医院：李南方、周玲、张德莲、姚晓光、洪静、索菲亚、曹梅；中国疾病预防控制中心：吴静、石文惠、翟屹、何柳。

参考文献

[1] Ammar KA, Redfield MM, Mahoney DW, et al. Central obesity: association with left ventricular dysfunction and mortality in the community [J]. Am Heart J, 2008, 156 (5): 975-981. DOI: 10.1016/j. ahj.2008.06.018.

[2] Dagenais GR, Yi Q, Mann JF, et al Prognostic impact of body weight and abdominal obesity in women and men with cardiovascular disease [J]. Am Heart J, 2005, 149(1): 54-60. DOI: 10.1016/j. ahj.2004.07.009.

[3] Gordon-Larsen P, Wang HJ, Popkin BM. Overweight dynamics in Chinese children and adults [J] Obes Rev, 2014, 15(1): 37-48. DOI: IO. IIII/obr.12121.

[4] Yamashita K. Kondo T, Osugi S, et al. The significance of measuring body fat percentage determined by bioelectrical impedance analysis for detecting subjects with cardiovascular disease risk factors [J]. Circ J, 2012, 76(10): 2435-2442. DOI: 10.1253/circj. CJ-12-0337.

[5] Cho YG, Song HJ, Kim JM, et al. The estimation of cardiovascular risk factors by body mass index and body fat percentage in Korean male adults[J]. Metabolism, 2009, 58 (6): 765-771. DOI: 10.1016a. metabol.2009.01.004.

[6] Zeng Q, Dong SY, Sun XN, et al. Percent body fat is a better predictor of cardiovascular risk factors than body mass index [J]. Braz J Med Biol Res, 2012, 45(7): 591-600. DOI: 10.1590/SOIOO-879X2012007500059.

[7] 董剩勇，王曼柳，孙晓楠，等．体脂肪率评估心血管危险因素研究 [J] 中国全科医学，2015, 18(36): 4416-4421. DOI: 10.3969/ j. issn.1007-9572.2015.36.004.

[8] Schuster J, Vogel P, Eckhardt C, et al. Applicability of the visceral adiposity index (VAI) in predicting components of metabolic syndrome in young adults [J]. Nutr Hosp, 2014, 30 (4): 806-812. DOI: 10.3305/ nh.2014.30.4.7644.

[9] 窦相峰，白真真，闫坤丽，等．女性内脏脂肪指数与代谢综合征的关系 [J]．中国循证心血管医学杂志，2013, 5 (1): 24-26. DOI: 10.3969/j.1674-4055.2013.01.009.

[10] Hyun YJ, Kim OY, Jang Y, et al. Evaluation of metabolic syndrome risk in Korean premenopausal women: not waist circumference but visceral fat [J]. Circ J, 2008, 72 (8): 1308-1315. DOI: 10.1253/circj .72.1308.

[11] Bosy-Westphal A, Later W, Hitze B. et al. Accuracy of bioelectrical impedance consumer devices for measurement ofbody composition in comparison to whole body magnetic resonance imaging and dual X-ray absorptiometry [J]. Obes Facts, 2008, 1(6): 319-324. DOI: 10.1159/000176061.

[12] Amlov J, Ingelsson E, Sundstrom J, et al. Impact of body mass index and the metabolic syndrome on the risk of cardiovascular disease and death in middle-aged men [J]. Circulation, 2010, 121 (2): 230-236. DOI: 10.1161/ circulationaha.109.887521.

[13] Yun JE, Won S, Sung J, et al. Impact of metabolic syndrome independent of insulin resistance on the development of cardiovascular disease [J]. Cire J.2012.76(10): 2443-2448. DOI: 10.1253/circj. CJ-12-0125.

[14] Lavie CJ, De Schutter A, Patel DA, et al. Body composition and survival in stable coronary heart disease: impact of lean mass index and body fat in the "obesity paradox" [J]. J Am Coll Cardiol, 2012, 60 (15): 1374-1380. DOI: 10.1016/j. j acc.2012.05.037.

[15] Tong J, Boyko EJ, Utzschneider KM, et al. Intra-abdominal fat accumulation predicts the development of the metabolic syndrome in non-diabetic Japanese-Americans [J]. Diabetologia, 2007, 50(6): 1156-1160. DOI: 10.1007/s00125-007-0651-y.

[16] Amato MC, Giordano C, Galia M, et al. Visceral adiposity index: a reliable indicator of visceral fat function associated with cardiometabolic risk [J]. Diabetes Care.2010.33 (4): 920-922. DOI: 10.2337/dc09-1825.

[17] WHO Expert Consultation. Appropriate body-mass index for Asian populations and its implications for policy and intervention strategies [J]. Lancet, 2004, 363 (9403): 157-163. DOI: 10.1016/s0140-6736(03) 15268-3.

[18] 郝光，王增武，张林峰等．不同肥胖测量指标对心脏代谢性疾病测价值的比较 [J]．医学研究杂志，2014, 43 (12): 18-22.

[19] Knowles KM, Paiva LL, Sanchez SE, et al. Waist circumference, body mass index, and other measures of adiposity in predicting cardiovascular disease risk factors among peruvian adults [J]. Int J Hypertens, 2011, 2011: 931402. DOI: 10.4061/2011/ 931402.

[20] 张强，陈晓平，施迪，等. 内脏脂肪指数与缺血性心血管病发病风险的关系 [J]. 西部医学，2016, 28 (lO): 1378-1381, 1385. DOI: 10.3969/j. issn.1672-3511.2016.10.010.

[21] Matsushita Y, Nakagawa T, Yamamoto S, et al. Associations of visceral and subcutaneous fat areas with the prevalence of metabolic risk factor clustering in 6 292 Japanese individuals : the Hitachi Health Study [J]. Diabetes Care, 2010, 33 (9) 2117-2119. DOI: 10.2337/dcl0-0120.

[22] Mathieu P, Pibarot P, Larose E, et al. Visceral obesity and the heart [J]. Int J Biochem Cell Biol, 2008, 40 (5): 821-836. DOI: 10.1016/j. biocel.2007.12.001.

[23] Amato MC, Giordano C, Pitrone M, et al. Cut-off points of the visceral adiposity index (VAI) identifying a visceral adipose dysfunction associated with cardiometabolic risk in a Caucasian Sicilian population [J]. Lipids Health Dis, 2011, 10: 183. DOI: 10.1186/1476-5llx-10-183.

西藏不同海拔地区高血压患病情况调查△

亢玉婷，王　馨，陈　祚，张林峰，董　莹，聂静雨，王佳丽，郑聪毅，邵　澜，田　野，王增武

中国医学科学院阜外医院，国家心血管病中心社区防治部　北京．102308

通讯作者：王增武，E-mail：wangzengwu@foxmail.com

摘　要　目的　了解西藏林芝县、堆龙德庆县与安多县 3 个不同海拔高度地区居民高血压患病状况，为高海拔地区高血压的防治提供依据。**方法**　于 2015～2016 年，采用分层多阶段随机抽样，在林芝县（3 000 m）、堆龙德庆县（3 600 m）和安多县（4 700 m）共调查 15 岁及以上人群 2 832 人。采用统一制作的问卷收集居民年龄、性别、血压、降高血压治疗等资料，并测量血压。用 2010 年第 6 次人口普查数据对年龄、性别进行率的标化。用 SAS 9.4 进行数据的统计分析。计数资料的组间比较用 χ^2 检验，计量资料的组间比较用方差分析，用 SNK 法进行两两比较。**结果**　林芝县、堆龙德庆县与安多县居民收缩压（SBP）分别为（126.1 ± 21.2）mmHg、（132.3 ± 22.4）mmHg 和（115.9 ± 17.9）mmHg，舒张压（DBP）分别为（77.4 ± 14.0）mmHg、（79.8 ± 14.0）mmHg 和（72.1 ± 13.7）mmHg，差异均有统计学意义（$P<0.01$）。正常高值血压患病率分别为 39.6 %、59.1% 和 21.5%，高血压患病率分别为 26.6%、34.2% 和 18.6%，差异均有统计学意义（χ^2 值分别为 186.43、54.47，$P<0.01$）；标化高血压患病率分别为 27.4%、30.0% 和 25.6%。**结论**　高海拔地区（4 700 m）血压水平、高血压患病率、正常高值血压患病率均较低。

关键词　高血压；西藏；患病率；现况调查

Investigation of hypertension morbidities at different altitudes of Tibet

Kang Yuting, Wang Xin, Chen Zuo, Zhang Linfeng, Dong Ying, Nie Jingyu, Wang Jiali, Zheng Congyi, Shao Lan, Tian Ye, Wang Zengwu

Division of Prevention and Community Health, National Center for Cardiovascular Diseases;

△　本文发表于：中国慢性病预防与控制，2017，25（6）：427-431.

Fuwai Hospital, PUMC and CAMS, Beijing 102308, China
Corresponding author: WANG Zeng-wu, E-mail: wangzengwu@foxmail. com

Abstract **Objective** To understand the hypertension morbidities of residents at different altitudes (Linzhi, Duilongdeqing and Anduo counties) of Tibet and to provide the basis for prevention and treatment of hypertension in high altitude areas. **Methods** From 2015 to 2016, the stratified multistage random sampling method was used to select 2 832 residents (≥ 15 years old) from Linzhi (altitude: 3 000 m), Duilongdeqing (altitude: 3 600 m) and Anduo (altitude: 4 700 m) counties. The specially designed questionnaire was used to collect the data of age, sex, antihypertension therapy and medical examination of blood pressure. The rates of hypertension were standardized by sex and age from 2010 population census data. The X^2 test, ANOVA and SNK method were used to analyze the data with SAS 9.4 software. **Results** The average SBP values of Linzhi, Duilongdeqing and Anduo counties were (126.1 ± 21.2), (132.3 ± 22.4) and (115.9 ± 17.9) mmHg, respectively; the average DBP values of Linzhi, Duilongdeqing, and Anduo counties were (77.4 ± 14.0), (79.8 ± 14.0), and (72.1 ± 13.7) mmHg, respectively; there were significant differences of SBP and DBP values among three counties ($P < 0.01$). The morbidities of normal high values for blood pressure were 39.6 %, 59.1%, and 21.5%, respectively; the morbidities of hypertension were 26.6%, 34.2%, and 18.6%, respectively; there were significant differences among three counties ($P < 0.01$). The standardized morbidities of hypertension were 27.4%, 30.0%, and 25.6%, respectively, in Linzhi, Duilongdeqing, and Anduo counties. **Conclusions** The blood pressure level, hypertension morbidity and morbidity of normal high values for blood pressure in highest altitude area (4 700 m) are lower.

Key words Hypertension; Tibet; Morbidity; Section investigation

高血压现已成为发展中国家主要的公共卫生问题[1]。研究显示，62% 的脑卒中与 49% 的心肌梗死发病与高血压有关[2]。最新研究亦显示，我国高血压患病率高达 25.6%[3]。西藏地处青藏高原，具有独特的地理特征和生活饮食习惯[4-5]。基于现有文献，关于西藏不同海拔高度高血压患病特点数据较为缺乏，仍需进一步研究。本文中通过对西藏林芝、拉萨以及那曲 3 个地区人群高血压患病情况的调查，探讨海拔高度与高血压的关系。

1. 对象与方法

1.1 对象

数据来源于公益性行业科研专项“西藏与新疆地区慢性心肺疾病现状调查研究”。于 2015 ~ 2016 年采用分层多阶段随机抽样方法，首先，在西藏进行城乡分层，在每层内采用成比例抽样法（PPS）抽取所需数量的区 / 县，然后，采用简单随机抽样法在被抽中的区 /

县中抽取2个街道或乡镇，在每个被抽中的街道或乡镇中采用简单随机抽样法抽取3个居委会或村委会，最后在被抽中的居委会或村委会中分性别、年龄采用简单随机抽样法随机抽取15岁及以上居民作为调查对象。共抽取6个区/县，每个区/县抽取1 000名调查对象。由于其他区/县数据仍在收集，本研究纳入林芝县（海拔3 000 m）、拉萨市堆龙德庆县（海拔3 600 m）和那曲安多县（海拔4 700 m）3个地区2 932人。排除年龄、性别、血压等重要变量数据不完整的对象，实际分析2 832人。本研究通过中国医学科学院阜外医院伦理委员会批准，所有调查对象均签署知情同意书。

1.2 方法

调查人群采用统一的调查方案、调查手册及调查问卷。各人群的主要调查人员、质控人员以及资料录入人员在调查前均进行培训并通过考核。问卷调查内容包括：（1）一般情况：姓名、性别、出生日期等。（2）高血压患病调查及高血压或糖尿病家族史、既往用药史、吸烟和饮酒等信息。（3）主要测量指标：包括身高、体重、腰围和血压等。其中，血压的测量应用Omron HBP-1300电子血压计。调查对象静坐休息5 min后，测量调查对象右上臂血压，连续测3次，每次至少间隔30 s，取3次血压的平均值作为调查对象的最终血压值。要求调查对象测量前半小时内避免吸烟、饮酒、饮用含有咖啡因的饮料以及剧烈运动。

1.3 相关定义与分类

高血压诊断标准采用《2010年中国高血压指南》[6]：收缩压（SBP）≥ 140 mmHg和/或舒张压（DBP）≥ 90 mmHg或正在服降压药者定义为高血压。正常高值血压为120 mmHg ≤ SBP < 140 mmHg和/或80 mmHg ≤ DBP < 90 mmHg。体重指数（BMI）= 体重（kg）/ 身高（m）^{2}。BMI ≥ 24 kg/m^{2}定义为超重或肥胖。腹型肥胖定义为：男性腰围≥ 90 cm，女性腰围≥ 85 cm[6]。吸烟者定义为一生中至少吸过20支且最近1个月仍在吸烟。饮酒定义为最近1个月每周至少饮酒1次。

1.4 统计学分析

用SAS 9.4进行数据的统计分析。计数资料用频数表描述分布，组间比较用χ^2检验，根据Bonferroni方法校正 α 进行两两比较；计量资料用$\bar{x}$ ± SD进行描述，组间比较用方差分析，用SNK法进行两两比较。用2010年第6次人口普查数据进行率的标化。检验水准 α = 0.05。

2. 结果

2.1 调查对象的人口学特征

堆龙德庆县人群平均年龄、腹型肥胖率较其他两个地区高，而高中及以上学历者所占比例低于其他两个地区，且两两比较，差异均有统计学意义（$P < 0.05$）。安多县超重或肥胖率及有高血压或糖尿病家族史的人群所占比例高于其他 2 个地区，差异均有统计学意义（$P<0.05$）。林芝县男性吸烟比例较其他两个地区高，差异均有统计学意义（$P<0.05$），见表 1。

2.2 不同海拔地区调查人群血压水平分布特点

林芝县、堆龙德庆县与安多县总人群 SBP 平均水平分别为（126.1 ± 21.2）、（132.3 ± 22.4）和（115.9 ± 17.9）mmHg，差异有统计学意义（$F = 147.00$，$P < 0.01$）。除高中及以上学历外，在其他各层安多县 SBP 水平均明显低于其他 2 个地区，差异均有统计学意义（$P < 0.05$）。堆龙德庆县女性及城镇户口人群 SBP 平均水平高于林芝县，差异有统计学意义（$P < 0.05$），见表 2。林芝县、堆龙德庆县与安多县总人群 DBP 平均水平分别为（77.4 ± 14.0）、（79.8 ± 14.0）、（72.1 ± 13.7）mmHg，差异有统计学意义（$F = 71.70$，$P < 0.01$）。安多县男性与腹型肥胖人群 DBP 水平明显低于其他 2 个地区，堆龙德庆县超重或肥胖与腹型肥胖人群 DBP 平均水平明显低于林芝县，差异均有统计学意义（$P < 0.05$），3 个地区吸烟与饮酒人群 DBP 水平比较，差异均无统计学意义（F 值分别为 0.73、2.54，$P > 0.05$）。3 个地区 SBP 与 DBP 水平均随着年龄增长而升高，见表 3。

表 1　西藏不同海拔地区人群一般特征

地区	性别		脉搏（次 /min，$\bar{x}$ ± SD）		年龄（岁，$\bar{x}$ ± SD）		城镇户口		高中及以上学历	
	男性	女性	男性	女性	男性	女性	男性	女性	男性	女性
林芝县	496	584	73.5 ± 10.8	73.5 ± 10.2	39.9 ± 17.0	41.6 ± 16.5	123（24.8）	38（6.5）	235（47.4）	133（22.8）
堆龙德庆县	267	471	77.2 ± 12.6[a]	77.9 ± 11.4[a]	46.8 ± 13.9[a]	46.7 ± 13.6[a]	2（0.8）[a]	5（1.1）[a]	7（2.6）[a]	19（4.0）
安多县	480	534	75.7 ± 12.7[a]	74.2 ± 12.0[b]	37.5 ± 14.8[b]	38.1 ± 14.7[ab]	275（57.3）[ab]	255（47.8）[ab]	158（32.9）[ab]	144（27.0）
χ^2 值或 F 值	F = 9.32	F = 22.38	F = 30.71	F = 41.76	χ^2 = 271.34	χ^2 = 449.60	χ^2 = 159.51	χ^2 = 97.30		
P 值	< 0.01	< 0.01	< 0.01	< 0.01	< 0.01	< 0.01	< 0.01	< 0.01		

地区	超重或肥胖		腹型肥胖		高血压或糖尿病家族史		吸烟		饮酒	
	男性	女性	男性	女性	男性	女性	男性	女性	男性	女性
林芝县	64（12.9）	81（13.9）	154（31.1）	147（25.2）	161（32.5）	203（34.8）	176（35.5）	8（1.4）	96（19.4）	34（5.8）
堆龙德庆县	51（19.1）	102（21.7）[a]	152（56.9）[a]	297（63.1）[a]	3（1.1）[a]	30（6.4）[a]	40（15.0）[a]	6（1.3）	12（4.5）[a]	10（2.1）
安多县	99（20.6）[a]	137（25.7）[a]	174（36.3）[b]	212（39.7）[ab]	209（43.5）[ab]	294（55.1）[ab]	117（24.4）[ab]	17（3.2）[ab]	43（9.0）[a]	10（1.9）
χ^2 值	11.50	25.05	50.98	155.22	149.34	268.96	39.53	6.40	43.37	16.57
P 值	< 0.01	< 0.01	< 0.01	< 0.01	< 0.01	< 0.01	< 0.01	< 0.01	< 0.01	< 0.01

注：与林芝县比较，[a]$P < 0.05$；与堆龙德庆县比较，[b]$P < 0.05$；括号外数据为例数，括号内数据为率（%）。

表 2　西藏不同海拔地区人群收缩压分布情况（$\bar{x}$ ± SD，mmHg）

地　区	性　别		年　龄			
	男性	女性	15～44 岁	45～54 岁	55～64 岁	65～岁
林芝县	127.3 ± 20.8	125.0 ± 21.5	117.1 ± 12.5	131.8 ± 20.3	142.0 ± 22.0	148.7 ± 27.3
堆龙德庆县	133.4 ± 19.8	131.6 ± 23.7^{a}	122.9 ± 15.0^{a}	133.3 ± 21.7	143.2 ± 24.5	152.6 ± 28.6
安多县	119.0 ± 17.0^{ab}	113.1 ± 18.2^{ab}	110.8 ± 12.4^{ab}	123.8 ± 20.8^{ab}	129.9 ± 22.2^{ab}	136.0 ± 25.1^{ab}
F 值	52.83	100.59	105.42	10.70	8.65	6.96
P 值	< 0.01	< 0.01	< 0.01	< 0.01	< 0.01	< 0.01

地区	城镇户口	高中及以上学历	超重或肥胖	腹型肥胖	家族史	吸烟	饮酒
林芝县	120.3 ± 14.2	115.8 ± 12.8	138.9 ± 22.7	136.1 ± 22.1	135.1 ± 24.5	126.7 ± 21.4	132.5 ± 21.3
堆龙德庆县	151.6 ± 35.6^{a}	118.8 ± 13.4	140.7 ± 23.6	135.6 ± 23.3	127.0 ± 21.5	132.1 ± 19.8	133.6 ± 18.3
安多县	118.9 ± 18.1^{b}	114.6 ± 13.8	126.2 ± 18.5^{ab}	123.0 ± 19.4^{ab}	116.4 ± 18.1^{ab}	119.4 ± 17.0^{ab}	121.3 ± 12.9^{ab}
F 值	12.20	1.60	27.36	44.25	38.69	9.08	6.98
P 值	< 0.01	0.20	< 0.01	< 0.01	< 0.01	< 0.01	< 0.01

注：与林芝县比较，$^{a}P < 0.05$；与堆龙德庆县比较，$^{b}P < 0.05$。

表 3　西藏不同海拔地区人群舒张压分布情况（$\bar{x}$ ± SD，mmHg）

地　区	性　别		年　龄			
	男性	女性	15～44 岁	45～54 岁	55～64 岁	65～岁
林芝县	78.6 ± 14.7	76.4 ± 13.3	71.8 ± 11.2	83.3 ± 13.1	87.8 ± 14.6	86.8 ± 13.3
堆龙德庆县	80.7 ± 12.9^{a}	79.2 ± 14.5^{a}	74.7 ± 11.7^{a}	81.2 ± 14.3	86.4 ± 13.0	86.7 ± 15.5
安多县	74.3 ± 14.3^{ab}	70.2 ± 12.8^{ab}	68.3 ± 11.3^{ab}	80.2 ± 14.2^{ab}	82.3 ± 12.8^{a}	83.5 ± 15.8
F 值	20.41	59.79	39.50	2.60	3.92	1.14
P 值	< 0.01	< 0.01	< 0.01	< 0.05	< 0.05	> 0.05

地区	城镇户口	高中及以上学历	超重或肥胖	腹型肥胖	家族史	吸烟	饮酒
林芝县	76.8 ± 11.0	70.0 ± 11.0	87.3 ± 13.4	84.6 ± 13.1	79.0 ± 14.4	78.8 ± 15.0	83.6 ± 14.2
堆龙德庆县	92.0 ± 17.0^{a}	72.2 ± 10.4	83.3 ± 14.6^{a}	81.4 ± 14.7^{a}	80.2 ± 16.3^{a}	78.1 ± 10.8	83.5 ± 11.8
安多县	75.7 ± 13.7^{b}	73.6 ± 11.3^{a}	80.4 ± 13.6^{a}	78.1 ± 13.6^{ab}	72.9 ± 14.1^{b}	76.9 ± 13.3	78.9 ± 11.0

续表

地区	城镇户口	高中及以上学历	超重或肥胖	腹型肥胖	家族史	吸烟	饮酒
F 值	5.54	8.67	11.01	19.00	20.81	0.73	2.54
P 值	< 0.01	< 0.01	< 0.01	< 0.01	< 0.01	> 0.05	> 0.05

注：与林芝县比较，$^aP < 0.05$；与堆龙德庆县比较，$^bP < 0.05$。

2.3 不同海拔地区人群高血压患病情况分布特点

林芝县、堆龙德庆县和安多县高血压粗患病率分别为 26.6%、34.2% 和 18.6%，差异有统计学意义（$x^2 = 54.47$，$P < 0.01$）；标化高血压患病率分别为 27.4%、30.0% 和 25.6%。3 个地区男性高血压患病率均高于女性。在男性饮酒与家庭史人群中，安多县高血压患病率低于堆龙德庆县，差异均有统计学意义（$P < 0.05$）；在超重或肥胖与腹型肥胖人群中，随着海拔的升高，高血压患病率下降（$P < 0.05$），见表 4。

2.4 不同海拔地区正常高值血压患病率分布特点

林芝县、堆龙德庆县和安多县正常高值血压患病率分别为 39.6 %、59.1% 和 21.5%，差异有统计学意义（$x^2 = 186.43$，$P < 0.01$）。3 个地区男性正常高值血压患病率均高于女性。在超重或肥胖与腹型肥胖人群中，安多县正常高值血压患病率低于其他 2 个地区，差异有统计学意义（$P < 0.05$）。在男性吸烟人群，女性 15 ~ 44 岁及糖尿病、高血压家庭史人群中，堆龙德庆县正常高值血压患病率高于林芝县和安多县，差异均有统计学意义（$P < 0.05$），见表 5。

3. 讨论

本文中通过研究西藏 3 个海拔高度（分别 3 000、3 600 和 4 700 m）高血压患病率，初步探究高血压与海拔高度的关系，为进一步高血压防治提供理论基础。本研究发现，不同海拔高度人群血压有所差异，安多县 SBP 与 DBP 平均水平最低，堆龙德庆县 SBP 与 DBP 水平高于林芝县，但在腹型肥胖、超重或肥胖人群中血压水平却明显较低，正常高值血压患病率低于堆龙德庆县与林芝县。同样，标化后林芝县、堆龙德庆县与安多县高血压患病率分别为 27.4%、30.0% 和 25.6%，安多县高血压患病率最低。

表 4　西藏不同海拔地区人群高血压患病率分布情况

地区	性别		男性年龄				女性年龄			
	男性	女性	15～44 岁	45～54 岁	55～64 岁	65～岁	15～44 岁	45～54 岁	55～64 岁	65～岁
林芝县	496	584	34（11.0）	34（39.1）	38（76.0）	36（73.5）	23（07.1）	48（35.0）	37（52.9）	37（68.5）
堆龙德庆县	267	471	24（20.2）	28（38.9）	22（51.2）[a]	23（69.7）	23（11.0）	54（39.7）	43（55.8）	35（71.4）
安多县	480	534	34（10.1）[b]	28（34.6）	17（53.1）	20（66.7）	22（05.9）	28（31.8）	22（52.4）	18（58.1）
X^2 值			8.94	0.45	7.34	0.43	5.09	1.53	0.19	1.54
P 值			＜0.01	0.80	＜0.05	0.81	0.08	0.46	0.91	0.46

地区	腹型肥胖		超重或肥胖		饮酒		家族史		合计	
	男性	女性	男性	女性	男性	女性[c]	男性[c]	女性	男性	女性
林芝县	68（44.2）	69（46.9）	35（54.7）	42（51.9）	43（44.8）	9（26.5）	55（34.2）	52（25.6）	142（28.6）	145（24.8）
堆龙德庆县	67（44.1）	117（39.4）	22（43.1）	45（44.1）	8（66.7）	4（40.0）	3（100.0）[a]	10（33.3）	97（36.3）	155（32.9）[a]
安多县	55（31.6）[ab]	63（29.7）[ab]	37（37.4）	48（35.0）[a]	12（27.9）[b]	1（10.0）	55（26.3）[b]	56（19.0）	99（20.6）[ab]	90（16.9）[ab]
X^2 值	7.26	11.41	4.75	6.13	6.82			5.17	22.23	34.87
P 值	＜0.05	＜0.01	0.09	＜0.05	＜0.05	0.30	0.01	0.08	＜0.01	＜0.01

注：与林芝县比较，$^aP<0.05$；与堆龙德庆县比较，$^bP<0.05$；[c] 使用 Fisher 精确检验；括号外数据为例数，括号内数据为患病率（%）。

表 5　西藏不同海拔地区人群正常高值血压患病率分布情况

地区	性别		男性年龄				女性年龄			
	男性	女性	15～44 岁	45～54 岁	55～64 岁	65～岁	15～44 岁	45～54 岁	55～64 岁	65～岁
林芝县	496	584	107（34.5）	34（39.1）	7（14.0）	8（16.3）	77（23.9）	49（35.8）	23（32.9）	8（14.5）
堆龙德庆县	267	471	67（56.3）	26（36.1）	14（32.6）	4（12.1）	95（45.5）[a]	46（36.0）	27（35.1）	8（16.3）
安多县	480	534	70（20.8）[b]	23（28.4）	8（25.0）	6（20.0）	35（9.4）[b]	18（20.5）[ab]	8（19.0）[ab]	5（16.1）
X^2 值			67.96	4.51	0.68	2.35	107.52	11.28	9.02	1.00
P 值			＜0.01	0.10	0.71	0.30	＜0.01	＜0.01	＜0.01	0.61

地区	腹型肥胖		超重或肥胖		吸烟		家族史		合计	
	男性	女性	男性	女性	男性	女性[c]	男性	女性	男性	女性
林芝县	60（39.0）	45（30.6）	20（31.3）	31（38.3）	46（26.1）	3（37.5）	48（29.8）	55（27.1）	156（31.5）	157（26.9）

续表

地区	腹型肥胖		超重或肥胖		吸烟		家族史		合计	
	男性	女性	男性	女性	男性	女性[c]	男性	女性	男性	女性
堆龙德庆县	60（39.5）	101（34.0）	24（47.1）	36（35.3）	17（42.5）[a]	3（50.0）	0（0.0）	13（43.3）[a]	111（41.6）[a]	176（37.4）[a]
安多县	51（29.3）[ab]	41（19.3）[ab]	35（35.4）	32（23.4）[ab]	25（21.4）[b]	1（5.9）	96（26.8）	34（11.6）[ab]	107（22.3）[ab]	66（12.4）[ab]
X^2 值	17.82	30.45	4.91	23.96	11.26		2.08	42.22	64.14	136.91
P 值	< 0.01	< 0.01	0.09	< 0.01	< 0.01	0.01	0.15	< 0.01	< 0.01	< 0.01

注：与林芝县比较，$^aP < 0.05$；与堆龙德庆县比较，$^bP < 0.05$；[c] 使用 Fisher 精确检验；括号外数据为例数，括号内数据为患病率（%）。

尽管安多县超重或肥胖、腹型肥胖及有高血压或糖尿病家族史人群比例较高，但其 SBP、DBP 水平处于最低水平。表明海拔可能影响血压水平，且与血压呈负相关，一项尼泊尔的高海拔居民高血压调查结果[7]与本文结果一致。早在 1986 年，有研究显示，居住在海拔 4 000 m 以上的居民高血压患病率较低[8]。2015 年印度一项研究亦发现，与居住在 2 600 ~ 3 700 m 海拔高度的居民相比，居住在海拔 4 000 ~ 4 900 m 的农村居民高血压患病率较低[9]。但一项对藏民的研究结果显示，高海拔可以降低儿童与青少年的血压水平，对成人没有影响[10]。关于西藏高血压患病率的系统综述亦发现，海拔每升高 100 m，高血压患病率增高 2%[11]。目前，关于海拔对血压的影响仍存在争议，相关机制较为复杂[12]。

有研究显示，长期暴露于低温环境，机体会通过一系列调控方式降低心率，防止血压上升，包括抑制交感神经活性、激活副交感神经、下调心脏 β 肾上腺受体[13-14]。本文中安多县调查人群心率低于堆龙德庆县可能与此相关。另外，海拔对血压的影响可能与种族的基因表达相关，高海拔地区藏民血降钙素相关基因与肾上腺髓质素的高表达与其血压下降有关[15]。但有研究认为，高原缺氧可能通过交感神经活性升高、肾素分泌增多等途径升高血压[11，16]。高海拔对交感神经与副交感神经活性的影响有待进一步研究。

本研究中，堆龙德庆县 SBP 与 DBP 水平高于林芝县，但在腹型肥胖、超重或肥胖人群水平却明显较低。研究表明，海拔 2 600 m 的印度农村居民高血压患病率（33.0%）略高于 3 700 m 的居民（27.8%），与本文结果相似。但本研究中，林芝县、堆龙德庆县与安多县调查日期分别为 5、10 ~ 11 和 8 月，堆龙德庆县气温较低。研究表明，与夏天相比，冬天人体血压约上升 5 mmHg 左右。虽然堆龙德庆县测量血压时室温保持在 20℃左右，但仍无法抵消外界长期低温对血压上升的影响。仍需更多研究探讨气温、基因、交感神经活动、海拔高度之间的交互作用，进一步揭示海拔对血压的影响。

本次调查中，安多县正常高值血压患病率也较低。目前，国内外关于高海拔地区正常高值血压患病率的调查较为缺乏。吉林省 18 ~ 79 岁人群正常高值血压患病率为 36.0%[15]。

但有研究显示，血压处于 120 ~ 129 mmHg/80 ~ 84 mmHg 和 130 ~ 139 mmHg/85 ~ 89 mmHg 的中年人群，10 年后发生高血压的风险分别为 45% 和 64%[6]，表明目前林芝县与堆龙德庆县居民高血压患病现状堪忧。

林芝县、堆龙德庆县与安多县标化高血压患病率分别为 27.4%、30.0% 和 25.6%，安多县高血压患病率最低。2015 年西藏 15 岁以上人群高血压粗患病率在 34.1% ~ 41.0% 之间 [4-5]。本次调查患病率略低，但高于国内高血压患病率（25.2%）[3]。印度高海拔地区高血压患病率在 27.8% ~ 33.0% 之间，亦高于其国内高血压患病率（29.8%）[17]。其与国内平均水平的差异受饮食、运动、教育水平等多种因素影响，需进一步控制上述混杂因素，从而揭示海拔对高血压的影响。

本调查结果提示，不同海拔高度血压水平有所差异，高海拔地区血压与高血压患病率偏低。由于本研究未收集调查对象在西藏居住时间、饮食和运动等情况，缺乏基因与蛋白质表达水平等数据，无法探究海拔对血压影响的作用机制，需更多相关研究验证海拔与血压的关系及作用机制。

致谢

感谢参与项目的所有专家及所有调查人员。协作组组成单位及主要调查人员：国家心血管病中心、中国医学科学院阜外医院：王增武、张林峰、陈祚、王馨、邵澜、郭敏、田野、赵天明、范国辉、董莹、聂静雨、王佳丽、郑聪毅、贾秀云、朱曼璐、王文、陈伟伟、高润霖；卫生部北京医院：郭岩斐、孙铁英、王玉霞、柴迪、马雅立、仝亚琪；中国人民解放军总医院：陈韵岱、冯斌、朱庆磊、周珊珊、刘杰、王晶、杨丽娜、杨瑛、段鹏；新疆维吾尔自治区人民医院：李南方、周玲、张德莲、姚晓光、洪静、索菲亚、曹梅；中国疾病预防控制中心：吴静、石文惠、翟屹、何柳。

参考文献

[1] Sule S, Tekin A, Yunus E, et al. Changes in hypertension prevalence, awareness, treatment, and control rates in Turkey from 2003 to 2012 [J]. J Hypertens, 2016, 34(6): 1208-1217.

[2] 胡大一，郭艺芳. 重视高血压的防治 [J]. 中国实用内科杂志，2009, 29(9): 781-782.

[3] 国家卫生计生委疾病预防控制局. 中国居民营养与慢性病状况报告 (2015 年)[R]. 北京：人民卫生出版社，2015.

[4] Huang XB, Zhou ZY, Liu JX, et al. Prevalence, awareness, treatment, and control of hypertension among China's Sichuan Tibetan population: a cross-sectional study [J]. Clin Exp Hypertens, 2016, 38(5): 457-463.

[5] Li X, Cai H, He J, et al. Prevalence, awareness, treatment and control of hypertension in Tibetan monks from Gansu Province, Northwest China [J]. Clin Exp Hypertens, 2015, 37(7): 536-541.

[6] 中国高血压防治指南修订委员会．中国高血压防治指南 2010 [J]．中华心血管病杂志，2011, 39(7): 579-616.

[7] Shrestha S, Shrestha A, Shrestha S, et al. Blood pressure in inhabitants of high altitude of Western Nepal [J]. JNMA J Nepal Med Assoc, 2012, 52(188): 154-158.

[8] Dasgupta DJ. Study of blood pressure of a high altitude community at Spiti (4 000 m)[J]. Indian Heart J, 1986, 38(2): 134-137.

[9] Norboo T, Stobdan T, Tsering N, et al. Prevalence of hypertension at high altitude: cross-sectional survey in Ladakh, NorthernIndia 2007-2011[J]. BMJ Open, 2015, 5(4): e007026.

[10] Tripathy V, Gupta R. Blood pressure variation among Tibetans at different altitudes [J]. Ann Hum Biol, 2007, 34(4): 470-483.

[11] Mingji C, Onakpoya IJ, Perera R, et al. Relationship between altitude and the prevalence of hypertension in Tibet: a systematic review [J]. Heart, 2015, 101(13): 1054-1060.

[12] Sizlan A, Ogur R, Ozer M, et al. Blood pressure changes in young male subjects exposed to a median altitude [J]. Clin Auton Res, 2008, 18(2): 84-89.

[13] Richalet JP, Larmignat P, Rathat C, et al. Decreased cardiac response to isoproterenol infusion in acute and chronichypoxia [J]. J Appl Physiol, 1988, 65(5): 1957-1961.

[14] Marshall JM. Peripheral chemoreceptorsand cardiovascular regulation [J]. Physiol Rev, 1994, 74(3): 543-594.

[15] 苏晓灵，周白丽，王嵘．不同海拔地区藏、汉族高血压患者血 CGRP、ADM 含量 [J]．青海医学院学报，2011, 32(2): 121-123.

[16] Bernardi L, Passino C, Wilmerding V, et al. Breathing patternsand cardiovascular autonomicmodulation during hypoxia induced by simulated altitude [J]. J Hypertensm, 2001, 19(5): 947-958.

[17] Anchala R, Kannuri NK, Pant H, et al. Hypertension in India: a systematic review and meta-analysis of prevalence, awareness, and control of hypertension [J]. J Hypertens, 2014, 32(6): 1170-1177.

系统聚类分析探讨老年人呼吸道疾病的临床表型△

宁　璞，郭岩斐，孙铁英，张洪胜，柴　迪，李晓梦

北京医院呼吸与危重症医学科，北京 100730

通信作者：郭岩斐，Email：yanfeiguo2003@126.com

摘　要　目的　采用系统聚类分析对老年呼吸道疾病患者的临床特征进行识别及分组，形成表型。**方法**　前瞻性纳入67例有喘息症状的老年患者，收集人口统计学资料、呼吸道症状、吸烟年数、急性加重情况、特应性症状、呼气峰流速日志等。患者于病情稳定期进行肺功能检查，并检测血清总IgE水平、外周血嗜酸性粒细胞计数，对患者进行系统聚类分析。**结果**　经系统聚类分析可将患者分为4类：①不吸烟、肺功能正常、血清总IgE升高、具有机体特应性的哮喘患者；②不吸烟、肺功能正常、仅有喘息症状的患者；③吸烟、重度气流受限、生活质量差的慢性阻塞性肺疾病（慢阻肺）患者；④吸烟、有气流受限、血清总IgE明显升高的哮喘－慢阻肺重叠综合征患者。4种表型患者在用药前第1秒用力呼气容积（FEV_1）/用力肺活量（FVC）、FEV_1/预计值、FEV，改善率和最大呼气中段流速（MMEF）/预计值、一氧化碳弥散系数（DLCO）/残气量（VA）/预计值、残气量（RV）/预计值、血清总IgE水平、累计吸烟量、圣乔治呼吸系统问卷（SGRQ）评分差异有统计学意义（$P<0.05$ 或 $P<0.01$）。**结论**　聚类分析可识别老年呼吸道疾病患者不同的临床表型，与单纯哮喘或慢阻肺患者相比，哮喘－慢阻肺重叠综合征患者肺功能下降明显，急性加重次数多，生活质量最差，需要引起重视。

关键词　呼吸道疾病；表型；聚类分析

Investigation of distinct clinical phenotypes of airways disease in the elderly based on hierarchical cluster analysis

Ning Pu, Guo Yanfei, Sun Tieying, Zhang Hongsheng, Chai Di, Li Xiaomeng

Department of Respiratory and Critical Care Medicine, Beijing Hospital, Beijing 100730, China

△　本文发表于：中华老年医学杂志，2016，35（3）：256-259.

Corresponding author: Guo Yanfei, Email: yanfeiguo2003@126. com

Abstract Objective To explore the clinical phenotype of airways disease in elderly patients using hierarchical cluster analysis. **Methods** A total of 67 elderly patients with respiratory symptoms were enrolled in a prospective study. Demographic and clinical data, such as respiratory symptoms, cumulative tobacco cigarette consumption, acute exacerbation, atopic symptoms and peak flow diary were collected. Pulmonary function tests, blood tests (total serum IgE level and blood eosinophil level) were performed in each patient during the stable stage. Then patients with different clinical phenotype were identified by hierarchical cluster analysis. **Results** Four clusters were identified with the following characteristics by hierarchical cluster analysis: cluster 1, atopic patients with no smoking, normal lung function, but increased total serum IgE levels and asthma symptom; cluster 2, patients with no smoking and normal pulmonary function with wheezing but without chronic cough; cluster 3, patients with chronic obstructive pulmonary disease and smoking, severe airflow limitation and poor quality of life; and cluster 4, patients with asthma-chronic obstructive pulmonary disease overlap syndrome and smoking, airflow limitation and increased total serum IgE levels. The forced expiratory volume in 1 second (FEV_1)/forced vital capacity(FVC)ratio, FEV_1/predicted value, rate of FEV_1 change, maximal mid-expiratory flow (MMEF)/predicted value, the diffusion lung capacity for carbon monoxide (DLCO)/alveolar volume (VA)/predicted value, residual volume (RV)/predicted value, total serum IgE levels, cumulative tobacco cigarette consumption, the St. George's Respiratory Questionnaire (SGRQ) score had significant differences in patients before versus after treatment (all $P < 0.05$ or $P < 0.01$). **Conclusions** Based on hierarchical cluster analysis, distinct clinical phenotypes of airways disease in elderly patients can be identified. With patients having asthma or COPD alone, patients with Asthma-COPD overlap syndrome (ACOS) always experience a more rapid decline in lung function and frequent exacerbations, having poor health-related quality-of-life (HRQOL) outcomes, which deserve our high attention.

Key words Respiratory trac diseases; Phenotype; Cluster analysis

呼吸道疾病如支气管哮喘、慢性阻塞性肺疾病（以下简称慢阻肺）、肺气肿等相互之间存在着重叠性[1]。近年来疾病的“表型”成为研究热点[2，3]，是指某一生物体特定的外观或组成部分，疾病分型的最终目标是为了发现具有独特预后或治疗特征的患者组别。对疾病的表型进行研究，有助于更加深入地认识疾病的异质性。目前国际上有很多研究致力于探索慢性阻塞性肺疾病、哮喘、肺气肿、呼吸道阻塞性疾病的表型，如 Gagnon 等[4]对全球慢性阻塞性肺病防治倡议（GOLD）1 级慢阻肺患者进行的表型研究，Cho 等[5]对肺气肿患者进行的聚类分析研究及 Haldar 等[6]对哮喘表型的研究等，对深入理解疾病特征和指导临床治疗都有很大帮助。

对于老年患者，典型的慢性支气管炎、哮喘和慢阻肺的鉴别并不困难。但临床上我们经常遇到一些老年哮喘患者，症状反复加重，逐渐出现固定的气流受限，呼吸道中有较多嗜酸性粒细胞和中性粒细胞浸润，呼吸道结构逐渐发生纤维化甚至肺泡结构破坏，给予糖皮质激素及 β 受体激动剂治疗后效果欠佳；另外，也有些不吸烟的老年慢阻肺患者，若呼吸道中嗜酸性粒细胞增多，则可能表现出部分可逆性的气流受限，给予糖皮质激素治疗疗效较好。因此，临床上对老年呼吸道疾病的诊断和鉴别存在一些困难，探究老年呼吸道疾病患者的临床表型对指导该类患者的个体化治疗尤为重要。

聚类分析主要是通过距离的远近与相似程度来判断个体之间是否有聚集现象，从而将研究对象分成不同的类别。聚类分析方法主要包括系统聚类、K 均值聚类、二阶段聚类法等。本研究通过收集具有喘息症状的老年患者的临床资料，采用系统聚类法来探索该类患者的临床表型。

1. 对象和方法

1.1 对象

前瞻性研究，选取 2013 ~ 2015 年北京市两个社区的居民作为受试对象，该研究通过北京医院伦理委员会批准，受试者均签署知情同意书。入选标准：①年龄 ≥ 60 岁；②过去 1 年内曾出现喘息症状（喘息定义为：静息状态下或活动时出现呼吸急促、呼吸困难）；③签署知情同意书。

排除标准：①因任何原因不能完成研究者；②确诊患有哮喘、慢阻肺、慢性支气管炎以外的呼吸系统疾病的患者及其他任何可引起喘息症状的疾病，如肺纤维化、慢性心力衰竭等；③已知患有活动性肺结核的患者。

资料完整者共 67 例，年龄 60 ~ 89 岁，平均（69.3 ± 7.0）岁。

1.2 方法

（1）问卷调查：①呼吸系统问卷：包括人口学信息、呼吸系统症状、既往病史、特应性症状（如过敏性皮炎、鼻炎）、吸烟史、生物燃料接触史、并发症等；②圣乔治呼吸系统问卷（St. George's Respiratory Questionnaire，SGRQ）。

（2）血液采集：采取每位受试者外周血，由我院检验科进行血嗜酸性粒细胞计数、血清总 IgE 水平测定。

（3）肺功能检查：每位受试者于病情稳定期进行用药前后肺通气及弥散功能检查，由我院肺功能室专业人员使用同一台肺功能仪（Master Screen Body，Jaeger，Germany）完成。支气管舒张试验于吸入沙丁胺醇 400 μg 15 min 后进行。

（4）呼气峰流速日志：每位受试者使用便携式呼气峰流速仪，于每日清晨和晚上固定时间分别进行 3 次呼气峰流速测定，计算 1 周内 PEF 变异率。

（5）系统聚类法对患者进行聚类：选取 9 个变量：①用药前第 1 秒用力呼气容积（FEV_1）/ 用力肺活量（FVC）；②用药前 FEV_1/ 预计值 %；③用药后 FEV_1 改善率；④残气量（RV）/ 预计值；⑤一氧化碳弥散系数（DLCO/VA）/ 预计值；⑥呼气峰流速（PEF）变异率；⑦血清总 IgE 水平；⑧累计吸烟量（包 / 年）；⑨呼吸道症状（咳嗽、咳痰）。

1.3 统计学方法

采用 SPSS 19.0 软件，选用以上 9 个变量，聚类方法选择组间联接法，度量标准为平方 Euclidean 距离。所有计量资料均用中位数（四分位数间距）表示，组间比较采用 Kruskal-Wallis 非参数秩和检验；计数资料如呼吸道症状、性别、特应性症状等，以率或百分数表示，组间比较采用 χ^2 检验，$P < 0.05$ 为差异有统计学意义。

2. 结果

2.1 受试者变量特征描述

表 1 层次聚类分析 4 种表型的样本特征

指　标	表型 1（12 例）	表型 2（13 例）	表型 3（21 例）	表型 4（21 例）	P 值
性别（男 / 女，例）	8/4	7/6	7/14	18/3	> 0.05
年龄（岁）*	71.0（60.0 ~ 82.0）	69.0（60.0 ~ 89.0）	70.0（61.0 ~ 84.0）	66.0（60.0 ~ 78.0）	> 0.05
药前 FEV_1/FVC（%）*	73.9（58.0 ~ 87.0）	71.0（66.5 ~ 84.3）	57.2（35.7 ~ 81.6）	61.3（29.1 ~ 87.0）	< 0.01
药前 FEV_1/ 预计值（%）*	86.5（62.0 ~ 118.5）	88.0（58.0 ~ 131.0）	50.0（21.3 ~ 90.0）	61.6（19.0 ~ 100.0）	< 0.01
药后 FEV_1 改善率（%）*	3.0（－1.0 ~ 26.0）	0.1（－20.0 ~ 6.0）	5.9（－6.1 ~ 26.0）	6.0（－4.2 ~ 30.0）	< 0.05
RV/ 预计值（%）*	89.0（82.0 ~ 105.0）	95.0（72.0 ~ 124.0）	144.0（127.0 ~ 188.0）	117.0（38.0 ~ 243.0）	< 0.01
DLCO/VA/ 预计值（%）*	93.4（72.3 ~ 102.1）	89.2（73.9 ~ 103.7）	66.7（50.7 ~ 99.3）	70.3（46.6 ~ 10.2）	< 0.01
PEF 变异率（%）*	19.1（11.2 ~ 39.8）	16.3（3.9 ~ 41.1）	17.3（1.3 ~ 55.1）	20.9（8.4 ~ 42.9）	> 0.05
MMEF/ 预计值（%）*	41.7（21.0 ~ 93.4）	49.3（26.0 ~ 139.0）	21.6（5.9 ~ 55.0）	30.0（5.0 ~ 100.0）	< 0.01
血清总 IgE（IU/ml）*	113.1（70.1 ~ 137.0）	17.1（5.0 ~ 70.2）	25.7（17.1 ~ 77.2）	299.0（156.0 ~ 1398.0）	< 0.01
血嗜酸性粒细胞	0.11（0.02 ~ 0.66）	0.12（0.05 ~ 0.39）	0.14（0.06 ~ 5.77）	0.15（0.00 ~ 0.61）	> 0.05
累计吸烟量（包 / 年）*	0（0 ~ 50.0）	0（0 ~ 44.0）	20.0（0 ~ 60.0）	30.0（0 ~ 120.0）	< 0.05

续表

指　标	表型 1（12 例）	表型 2（13 例）	表型 3（21 例）	表型 4（21 例）	P 值
呼吸道症状〔例（%）〕	4（33.3）	2（15.4）	7（33.3）	9（42.9）	>0.05
过敏性皮炎〔例（%）〕	6（50.0）	5（38.5）	10（47.6）	7（33.3）	>0.05
鼻炎〔例（%）〕	6（50.0）	7（53.8）	13（61.9）	6（28.6）	>0.05
SGRQ 评分（分）*	15.1（7.0 ~ 25.4）	19.1（7.5 ~ 43.7）	31.5（9.1 ~ 71.9）	29.9（6.1 ~ 55.7）	<0.01
1 年内加重〔例（%）〕	2（16.7）	2（15.4）	6（28.6）	3（14.3）	>0.05

注：* 中位数（四分位数间距）；FEV_1：第 1 秒用力呼气容积，FVC：用力肺活量，RV：残气量，DLCO/VA：一氧化碳弥散系数，PEF：呼气峰流速，MMEF：最大呼气中段流速，SGRQ：圣乔治呼吸系统问卷。

67 例患者用药前 FEV_1/FVC% 为（64.2 ± 13.3）%，FEV_1/ 预计值（69.4 ± 25.9）%，1 周内 PEF 变异率为（20.5 ± 10.0）%，血清总 IgE 为（166.8 ± 244.8）IU/ml，累计吸烟量（20.7 ± 23.3）包 / 年，22 例（32.8%）有慢性咳嗽、咳痰症状。

2.2　系统聚类分析

系统聚类分析结果显示，患者可分为 4 类，分别为 12、13、21、21 例，各类患者的特征见表 1。

对 4 种表型间各类指标进行比较结果显示，患者在用药前 FEV_1/FVC%、用药前 FEV_1/ 预计值、用药后 FEV_1 改善率、最大呼气中段流速（MMEF）/ 预计值、DLCO/VA/ 预计值、RV/ 预计值、血清总 IgE 水平、累计吸烟量、SGRQ 评分差异有统计学意义（$P < 0.05$ 或 $P < 0.01$），年龄、外周血嗜酸性粒细胞计数、性别、过敏性皮炎、鼻炎、PEF 变异率、呼吸道症状、1 年内加重次数差异无统计学意义（$P > 0.05$）。

第一类患者肺通气功能、弥散功能均良好，不吸烟，生活质量好，但血清总 IgE 升高，患过敏性皮炎、鼻炎的比例较高；第二类患者肺通气功能、弥散功能也均良好，血清总 IgE 正常，生活质量好，无吸烟史，仅具有喘息症状；第三类患者存在严重气流阻塞，肺通气功能、弥散功能均差，吸烟史较长，一年内急性加重比例高，生活质量差，血清总 IgE 正常；第四类患者肺通气、弥散功能均下降，吸烟史长，血清总 IgE 明显升高，咳嗽、咳痰症状重，生活质量差。

3. 讨论

本研究通过对过去 1 年内有喘息症状的老年人群进行聚类分析研究发现了不同的临床表型。第一类患者肺功能正常，IgE 升高，机体特应性高，具有哮喘的临床特点；第二类患者肺功能正常，仅有喘息症状；第三类患者属于重－极重度慢阻肺人群；第四类患者属于哮喘－慢阻肺重叠综合征表型，这一表型的患者发病率随年龄增长而升高，同时具有支气管哮喘和慢阻肺的特征，肺功能表现为不完全可逆的气流受限，伴有呼吸道高反应性，与支气管哮喘或慢阻肺相比，病情进展更快，临床症状更重，急性发作次数更多，生活质量低下，且预后较差。

我们的研究发现同样具有喘息症状的人群中，肺功能可能完全正常，也可能重度降低；机体特应性可能正常，也可能升高；吸烟史长短不一；临床症状轻重不等。因此研究呼吸道疾病表型有助于指导临床医生对患者提供个体化治疗。对于有喘息症状的老年患者，在除外心脏疾病以及肺间质纤维化、肺栓塞等其他可能引起喘息的病因后，应全面收集患者吸烟史、机体特应性、临床症状、肺功能、X 线胸片、胸部 CT、呼出气一氧化氮测定等指标，对患者的呼吸道炎症类型及病情轻重进行正确评估，据此选择合理的治疗。研究结果表明，呼吸道嗜酸性粒细胞炎症较重的慢阻肺患者可能需要增加吸入性糖皮质激素的剂量，甚至需要使用全身激素，肺气肿表型患者对吸入性糖皮质激素的反应较差，而使用长效 β2 激动剂、长效抗胆碱能药物、肺减容手术等却可得到较好的治疗效果。

系统聚类法主要通过距离的远近逐渐将所有的数据聚为一类，同一类中的对象有很大的相似性，而不同类间的对象则有很大的差异性。本研究中系统聚类的样本间的聚类过程为，每个样本有 9 个变量，则每个样本均为九维空间中的一个点，67 个样本就是九维空间的 67 个点，首先计算两个样本之间的距离，将距离最近的样本归为一类，再计算该类与剩余各类的距离，找到距离最近的两类再合并为新的一类，重复上述过程，直到将所有样本聚类。近年来聚类分析这种方法在呼吸系统疾病中已得到广泛应用[7-9]。在今后的疾病表型研究中，无论是临床表型、遗传学表型或是影像学表型，都可将聚类分析作为一种统计方法对疾病进行分型。

但是本研究也存在着一些不足之处。呼出气一氧化氮是反映机体特应性及呼吸道炎症类型的一个指标[10, 11]，但本研究因条件的限制未能纳入这类指标；胸部高分辨率 CT 目前已被广泛应用于肺气肿、气体陷闭和呼吸道壁厚度的定量评价，可通过观察肺部结构的改变来预测患者治疗反应及预后[12-14]，但本研究缺乏影像学资料。因此，开展大规模老年呼吸道疾病患者的表型研究，收集充分反映这类疾病病理生理学特征、临床特点的变量，将对识别表型更有帮助，这值得我们今后进一步加以探索。

参考文献

[1] Weatherall M, Travers J, Shirtcliffe PM, et al. Distinct clinical phenotypes of airways disease defined by cluster analysis[J]. Eur Respir J, 2009, 34 (4): 818-888. DOI: 10.1183/09031936.00174408.

[2] Garcia Aymerich J, Agusti A, Barbera JA, et al. Phenotypic heterogeneity of chronic obstructive pulmonary

disease [J]. Arch Bronconeumol, 2009, 45(3): 129-138. DOI: 10.1016/S1579-2129(09)70790-6.

[3] Kaneko Y, Masuko H, Sakamoto T, et al. Asthma phenotypes in Japanese adults-their associations with the CCL5 and ADRB2 Genotypes [J]. Allergol Int.2013, 62(1): 113-121. DOI: 10.2332/allergolint.12-OA-0467.

[4] Gagnon P, Casaburi R, Saey D, et al. Cluster analysis in patients with GOLD 1 chronic obstructive pulmonary disease [J]. PLoS One, 2015, 23(4): e0123626. DOI: 10.1371/journal. pone.0123626.

[5] Cho MH, Washko GR. Hoffmann TJ, et al. Cluster analysis in severe emphysema subjects using phenotype and genotype data: an exploratory investigation [J]. Respir Res, 2010, 11(5): 30. DOI: 10.1186/1465-9921-11-30.

[6] Haldar P, Pavord ID。Shaw DE, et al. Cluster analysis and clinical asthma phenotypes [J]. Am J Respir Crit Care Med, 2008, 178(3): 218-224. DOI: 10.1164/rccm.200711-1754OC.

[7] Vavougios GD, Natsios G, Pastaka C, et al. Phenotypes of comorbidity in OSAS patients: combining categorical principal component analysis with cluster analysis [J]. J Sleep Res, 2015, 25(1): 31-38. DOI: 10.1111/jsr.12344.

[8] Schatz M, Hsu JW, Zeiger RS, et al. Phenotypes determined by cluster analysis in severe or difficult-to-treat asthma [J]. J Allergy Clin Immunol, 2014, 133(6): 1549-1556. DOI: 10.1016/j. jaci.2013.10.006.

[9]Sakagami T, Hasegawa T, Koya T, et al. Cluster analysis identifies characteristic phenotypes of asthma with accelerated lung function decline [J]. J Asthma, 2014, 51(2): 113-118. DOI: 10.3109/02770903.2013.852201.

[10] Romero KM, Robinson CL, Baumann LM, et al. Role of exhaled nitric oxide as a predictor of atopy [J]. Respir Res, 2013, 14(5): 48. DOI: 10.1186/1465-9921-14-48.

[11] Tamada T, Sugiura H, Takahashi T, et al. Biomarker-based detection of asthma-COPD overlap syndrome in COPD populations [J]. Int J Chron Obstruct Pulmon Dis, 2015, 10(9): 2169-2176. DOI: 10.2147/COPD.

[12] Lee JS, Huh JW, Chae EJ, et al. Response patterns to bronchodilator andquantitative computed tomography in chronic obstructive disease [J]. Clin Physiol Funct Imaging, 2012, 32(1): 12-18. DOI: 10.1111/j.1475-097X.2011.01046. x.

[13] Bafadhel M, Umar I, Gupta S, et al. The role of CT scanning in multidimensional phenotyping of COPD[J]. Chest, 2011, 140(3): 634-642. DOI: 10.1378/chest.10-3007.

[14] Pike D, Kirby M, Eddy RL, et al. Regional heterogeneity of chronic obstructive pulmonary disease phenotypes: pulmonary 3He magnetic resonance imaging and computed tomography [J]. COPD, 2016, 20(1): 1-9.

肺间质纤维化合并肺气肿综合征的临床特点研究△

谭晓明[1]，郭岩斐[1]，张　旻[2]，杨菁菁[1]，孙铁英[1]*

1. 北京医院 / 国家老年医学中心呼吸与危重症医学科，北京 100730；
2. 北京医院 / 国家老年医学中心放射科，北京 100730
* 通信作者，Email：suntieying3@hotmail.com

摘　要　目的　探讨肺间质纤维化合并肺气肿（combined pulmonary fibrosis and emphysema，CPFE）综合征的临床特点。**方法**　收集本院 2000 年 1 月至 2016 年 1 月 CPFE 综合征住院患者资料，分析其临床资料、影像学、肺功能、血气分析和病情转归。**结果**　共纳入 55 例 CPFE 综合征患者。38 例有吸烟史。12 例患者在诊断 CPFE 综合征后出现肺癌。28 例死亡。7 例进行了尸体解剖，肺上叶的病理表现均为小叶中心型肺气肿和肺大泡，肺下叶 6 例为机化性肺炎，1 例为普通型间质性肺炎。16 例患者有肺动脉高压。肺功能指标：FVC%Pre（88.83 ± 22.42）%；FEV_1%Pre（79.52 ± 20.94）%；FEV_1/FVC%（67.87 ± 12.87）%；TLC%Pre（105.43 ± 27.91）%；RV/TLC%（49.8 ± 11.24）；DLCO%Pre（72.54 ± 27.66）。HRCT：肺气肿以小叶中心型为主，肺大泡 15 例，间隔旁肺气肿 11 例，平均肺气肿积分 2.86 ± 2.86；肺纤维化以网格影表现为主，平均肺纤维化积分 2.31 ± 1.56。DLCO 与吸烟量（$r=-0.324$，$P=0.016$），$PA\text{-}aO_2$（$r=-0.317$，$P=0.018$），RV/TLC%（$r=-0.293$，$P=0.03$），肺气肿积分（$r=-0.412$，$P=0.002$）各指标负相关。**结论**　CPFE 综合征是一种独立的疾病，吸烟是发病的重要因素；易出现肺动脉高压及肺癌；肺容积相对正常或者轻度下降，弥散能力显著下降且与影像学上肺气肿和肺纤维化所占比例相关。

关键词　肺纤维化；肺气肿；肺功能

Research of Combined Pulmonary Fibrosis and Emphysema

Tan Xiaoming[1], Guo Yanfei[2], Zhang Min[2], Yang Jingjing[2], Sun Tieying[2*]

1. Department of Respiratory and Critical Care Medicine, 2. Department of Radiology, Beijing Hospital, Beijing 100730, China

*Corresponding author, Email: suntieying3@hotmail. corn

△　本文发表于：中国医刊，2017，52（11）：17-22.

Abstract Objective To retrospectively analyse the clinical features, smoking history, pulmonary function, pulmonary artery pressure, mortality, and radiological appearance in patients with combined pulmonary fibrosis and emphysema (CPFE). **Method** We selected hospitalized patients since 2000 to 2016 at Beijing Hospital who had full information. Patients were diagnosed with CPFE according to the chest high-resolution computed tomography (HRCT) findings (with both emphysema of the upper zones and diffuse parenchymal lung disease with fibrosis of the lower zones of the lungs). We reviewed the clinical features, smoking history, pulmonary function, pulmonary artery pressure, mortality, and radiological appearance in these three different groups. **Result** Totally 55 CPFE cases were enrolled in this study. All patients but one were males. Age of this group was (84.11 ± 11.00) years. There were 38 smokers, and the smoking index was (24.39 ± 20.28) pack-years. Dyspnoea was presented in 41 patients and basal crackles were heard in 43 patients. Sixteen patients were admitted to the hospital as pulmonary fibrosis, while 39 patients as COPD. Twelve patients came to pass lung cancer and the mean time from diagnosis of CPFE to cancer was (3.56 ± 2.99) years. Finally, 28 patients died and the main reason was sepsis shock.7 autopsy cases showed centrilobular emphysema and bullae at the upper zone, while organized pneumonia at the lower zone. Only one case was UIP. Pulmonary hypertension [(59.31 ± 11.79) mmHg] was present in 29.1% of patients. Blood gas analysis (mean ± SD): PaO_2 (67.58 ± 13.26) mmHg; $PaCO_2$, (38.75 ± 8.7) mmHg; PA-aO_2, (58.76 ± 51.18) mmHg. Pulmonary function tests were as follows: FVC%Pre, (88.83 ± 22.42)%; FEV_1%Pre, (79.52 ± 20.94)%; FEV_1/FVC%, (67.87 ± 12.87)%; TLC%Pre, (105.43 ± 27.91)%; RV/TLC%, (49.8 ± 11.24); DLCO%Pre, (72.54 ± 27.66). **Conclusions** CPFE syndrome is a distinct clinical entity. Smoking is the principal risk factor for CPFE. Most of the patients have dyspnoea. A high prevalence of pulmonary artery hypertension and lung cancer is seen in CPFE syndrome. Patients with CPFE syndrome can present with a normal or nearly normal lung volume but a remarkable impairment in gas exchange and has a correlation with the proportion of emphysema and Pulmonary fibrosis on HRCT.

Key words Emphysema; pulmonary fibrosis; lung function

肺间质纤维化及肺气肿在病理上是相互独立、不能共存的两种疾病。然而，早在 1985 年 Nakata 等 [1] 就发现肺气肿患者的胸部 CT 中存在肺间质纤维化。1990 年 Wiggins 等 [2] 的研究证明了确诊为肺间质纤维化的患者中有上肺肺气肿的存在。2005 年，Cottin 等 [3] 报道了多个医学研究中心的共 61 例肺间质纤维化合并肺气肿病例，是目前为止报道例数最多的研究，提出这是一种独立的疾病，命名为肺间质纤维化合并肺气肿（combined pulmonary fibrosis and emphysema，CPFE）综合征。

CPFE 综合征在临床上并不少见，我国早在 1990 年季蓉等 [4] 就曾报告了 11 例肺气肿合并肺间质纤维化病例。2010 年彭敏等 [5] 探讨了 8 例 CPFE 综合征患者，其肺功能表现为肺容积相对正常而弥散功能显著下降。

CPFE 综合征由于双重的病理损伤造成肺的通气与换气功能严重障碍，临床表现为反复下呼吸道感染和逐渐加重的呼吸困难（容易被误诊为心力衰竭等），常合并肺动脉高压，预后差。本文旨在研究 CPFE 综合征的临床特点，以提高对此病的认识。

1. 对象和方法

1.1 对象

自 2000 年 1 月至 2016 年 1 月本院住院人群中选择本研究对象。高分辨 CT（HRCT）同时存在肺气肿及肺间质纤维化。肺气肿：边界清楚的低密度影，无壁或薄壁（$< 1mm$），或肺大泡（直径 $> 1cm$），病变以上肺野为主；肺间质纤维化：肺外周和下肺野为主的网格影和蜂窝肺，牵张性支气管扩张，可有局部、少量的磨玻璃影和（或）实变影。排除标准：结缔组织病相关性间质性肺疾病、药物性肺病、尘肺、结节病、外源性过敏性肺炎、肉芽肿性多血管炎、肺泡蛋白沉积症、慢性嗜酸细胞性肺炎。

1.2 方法

收集纳入本研究的 CPFE 患者的年龄、性别、吸烟（用吸烟包年数表示吸烟量，吸烟包年数 = 每日吸烟支数 /20 支 × 吸烟年数）、症状、体征、病程、基础疾病、病情演变及转归、尸检资料、肿瘤标志物、血气分析、心脏彩色多普勒超声、肺功能一秒用力呼气容积（forced expiratory volume in one second，FEV_1）、用力肺活量（forced vital capacity，FVC）、FEV_1/FVC、肺总量（total lung capacity，TLC）、残气量 / 肺总量比值（RV/TLC）、一氧化碳弥散量（DLCO）及各指标占预计值的百分比（%pre）等临床资料。

1.2.1 肺气肿指标的测量 采用视觉评分法（emphysematous visual scoring，EVS）[6]。双肺分别取 5 个层面（隆突上 6 cm、隆突上 3 cm、隆突、隆突下 3 cm 和隆突下 6 cm），评估各层面肺气肿程度分级（0 ~ 3 级）和范围分级（1 ~ 4 级），将各层面二者的乘积相加，再除以扫描层数。0 分为无肺气肿；0.1 ~ 8 分为轻度；8.1 ~ 16 分为中度；16.1 ~ 24 分为重度。

2.2.2 肺间质纤维化指标的测量 取主动脉弓上缘、隆突、膈肌上 1cm 水平，分别计算 3 个层面纤维化占相应肺野面积的百分比。分别计算磨玻璃影、小叶间隔增厚、网格影、蜂窝状影累计范围进行评分。0 分：无异常改变，1 分：累计范围在 1% ~ 25%；2 分：26% ~ 50%；3 分：51% ~ 75%；4 分：75% ~ 100%。将肺间质改变评分相加 [7]。

1.3 统计学处理

应用统计软件 SPSS 16.0 进行统计分析，计量数据以均数 ± 标准差表示，所有数据评价正态性分布，并与 DLCO 进行相关性比较，正态分布数据采用 Pearson 相关分析，非正态分布的数据采用非参数检验的等级相关分析。

2. 结果

2.1　一般资料

本研究共纳入研究对象 55 例，男性 54 例，女性 1 例，平均年龄（84.11 ± 11.00）岁。38 例有吸烟史。1 例患者出现咯血。16 例以肺间质纤维化（既往未诊断过肺气肿 /COPD）入院，39 例以肺气肿 /COPD 为首发疾病入院（表 1）。合并 3 种及以上基础疾病者 28 例。2 例患者在诊断时合并肺栓塞。9 例有肿瘤病史。8 例存在消化性溃疡。5 例有睡眠呼吸暂停综合征（表 2）。

表 1　55 例肺纤维化合并肺气肿综合征患者一般资料

项　目	例数（%）或均数 ± 标准差（范围）
年龄（岁）	84.11 ± 11.00（55 ~ 100）
性别（男 / 女）	54/1
吸烟（是 / 否）	38/17
吸烟量（包年）	24.39 ± 20.28（0 ~ 60）
活动后呼吸困难	41（74.5%）
咳嗽	38（69.1%）
咳痰	35（63.6%）
杵状指（趾）	9（16.4%）
下肺爆裂音	43（78.2%）

表 2　55 例肺纤维化合并肺气肿综合征患者基础疾病情况

疾病名称	例数（%）
糖尿病	12（21.8%）
高血压	37（67.3%）
冠心病	30（54.5%）
血脂异常	17（30.9%）
反流性食管炎	10（18.2%）
慢性胃炎	22（40.0%）

续表

疾病名称	例数（%）
慢性肾脏病	17（30.9%）
甲状腺疾病（包括甲状腺结节）	22（40.0%）

7 例从 HRCT 上表现出病情进展，肺间质纤维化进展 2 例，肺气肿 / 肺大泡进展 3 例（其中 1 例患者于半年后诊断为肺腺癌），1 例患者同时存在肺气肿和肺间质纤维化的进展。

28 例死亡，因“肺炎，感染中毒性休克”死亡占多数（表 3）。7 例进行了尸体解剖，尸检显示肺上叶的病理表现均为小叶中心型肺气肿和肺大泡，肺下叶的病理主要表现为机化性肺炎（6 例），仅 1 例为普通型间质性肺炎。

表 3　肺纤维化合并肺气肿综合征患者死亡原因（n = 28）

死亡原因	例数（%）
感染中毒性休克	13（46.4%）
急性呼吸窘迫综合征	5（17.9%）
上消化道出血	4（14.3%）
心源性休克	2（7.1%）
脑出血 / 脑疝	4（14.3%）

12 例患者在诊断后出现肺癌，从诊断到发生肺癌平均（3.56 ± 2.99）年。肺癌病理类型 5 例鳞癌，3 例腺癌，1 例小细胞肺癌，3 例未明确病理类型（PET-CT 提示肺癌）。40 例有肿瘤标志物升高，其中 26 例癌胚抗原（CEA）升高，18 例鳞状细胞癌相关抗原（SCC）升高，5 例神经元特异性烯醇酶（NSE）升高，18 例细胞角蛋白片段（CYFRA）升高（表 4）。

表 4　肺纤维化合并肺气肿综合征患者血清肿瘤标志物 ($\bar{x} \pm SD$)

肿瘤标志物	检测结果
CEA（ng/ml）（n = 26）	13.73 ± 13.68
SCC（ng/ml）（n = 18）	4.32 ± 4.10
NSE（ng/ml）（n = 5）	22.04 ± 2.76
CYFRA（ng/ml）（n = 18）	8.07 ± 4.70

40 例有低氧血症，18 例 I 型呼吸衰竭，8 例有二氧化碳潴留。静息不吸氧状态下血气分

析：PaO_2 34.4～95.6（67.58 ± 13.26）mmHg；$PaCO_2$ 23～72.5（38.75 ± 8.7）mmHg；PA-aO_2 14.4～337.7（58.76 ± 51.18）mmHg。

心脏彩色多普勒超声显示4例右室扩大。16例有肺动脉高压41～79 mmHg，平均（59.31 ± 11.79）mmHg。

阻塞性通气功能障碍22例，限制性通气功能障碍11例，混合型通气功能障碍6例，弥散功能障碍36例（表5）。28例患者的FEV1/FVC < 70%，占总例数51%。其中FEV1占预计值% < 50%者1例，50%～79%者18例，> 80%者9例。

2.2 胸部高分辨CT检查

肺气肿表现以小叶中心型为主，肺大泡15例，间隔旁肺气肿11例。肺纤维化以网格影表现为主，磨玻璃影也较常见，纵隔淋巴结肿大者15例。EVS评分0.2～11.4，平均2.86 ± 2.86。肺纤维化积分1～7，平均2.31 ± 1.56（表6）（图1、图2）。

表5 55例肺纤维化合并肺气肿综合征患者肺功能指标检测结果（$\bar{x}$ ± SD）

项目	检测结果
FVC（L）	2.75 ± 0.7
FVC占预计值%	88.83 ± 22.42
FEV_1（L）	1.83 ± 0.47
FEV_1占预计值%	79.52 ± 20.94
FEV_1/FVC%	67.87 ± 12.87
TLC（L）	5.75 ± 1.56
TLC占预计值%	105.43 ± 27.91
RV/TLC%	49.80 ± 11.24
DLCO（mL/mmHg/min）	11.08 ± 3.93
DLCO占预计值%	72.54 ± 27.66

表6 肺纤维化合并肺气肿综合征患者高分辨率CT肺纤维化表现

特　点	例　数	总　分
小叶间隔增厚	8	18
磨玻璃影	24	33
网格影	47	73
蜂窝肺	8	16

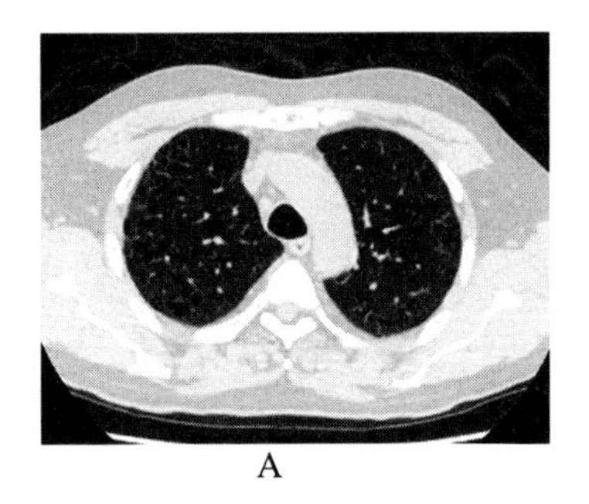
A

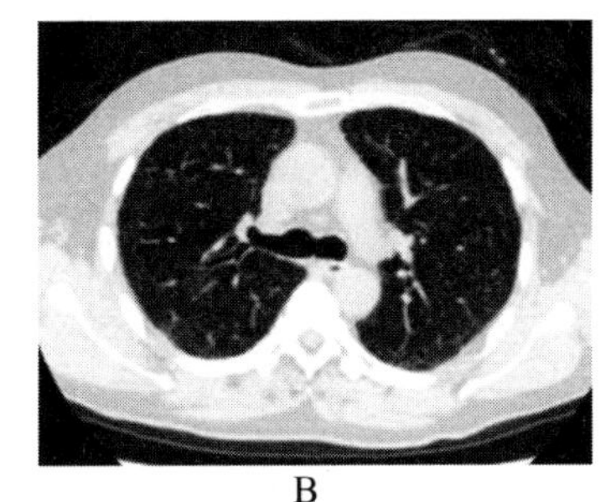
B

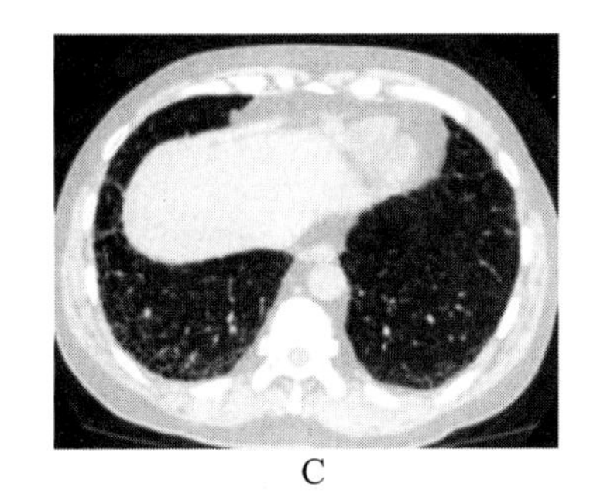
C

图 1　男性，58 岁，胸部 CT 薄层肺窗，两上肺小叶中心型肺气肿，下肺网格影及蜂窝；A）隆突上 3cm 层面两上肺小叶中心型肺气肿，无间质纤维化征象，视觉评分：受累范围 1 级，受累程度 1 级，评分为 1 分；B）隆突水平，小叶中心型肺气肿，视觉评分：受累范围 1 级，受累程度 1 级，评分为 1 分，两肺背侧胸膜下少许网格影，评分 1 分；C）膈肌上层面，网格影及蜂窝，受累范围 < 25%，评分 1 分

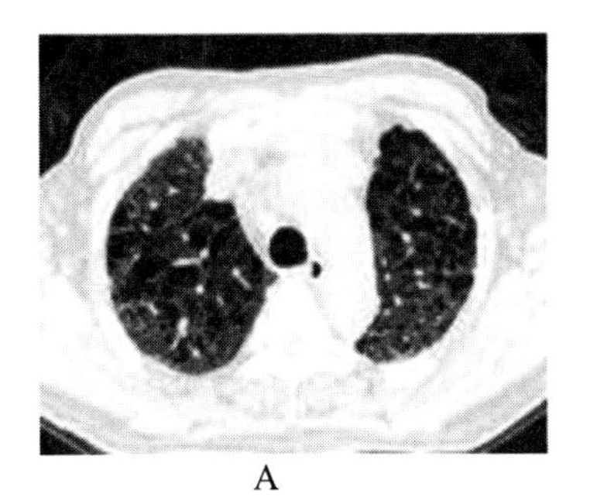
A

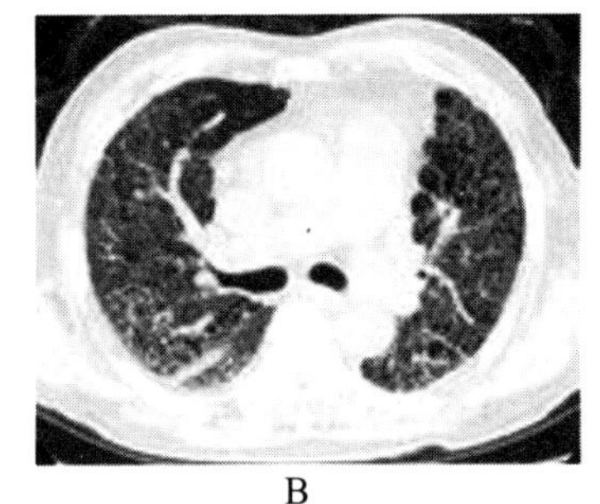
B

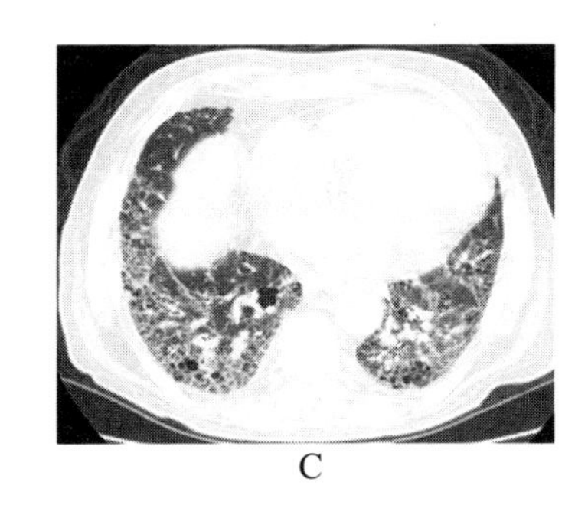
C

图 2　男性，78 岁，胸部 CT 薄层肺窗，两上肺小叶中心型肺气肿，下肺网格影及蜂窝；A）隆突上 3cm 层面，两上肺小叶中心型肺气肿，少许小叶间隔增厚。视觉评分：受累范围 2 级，受累程度 3 级，评分为 6 分；B）隆突水平，小叶中心型肺气肿。视觉评分受累范围 2 级，受累程度 2 级；两肺胸膜下网格影，评分 1 分；C）膈肌上层面网格影及蜂窝改变，评分 2 分，磨玻璃影，评分 2 分

2.3　各项指标与 DLCO 的相关性

吸烟量越大，肺气肿积分越高，其 DLCO 下降越明显。DLCO 与吸烟（$r = -0.324$，$P = 0.016$），肺气肿积分（$r = -0.412$，$P = 0.002$），$PA\text{-}aO_2$（$r = -0.317$，$P = 0.018$），RV/TLC%（$r = -0.293$，$P = 0.03$）各指标负相关（表 7）。

表 7　各项指标与一氧化碳弥散量的相关性

项　　目	相关系数 r/t	*P*
吸烟（包年）	－0.324	0.008
戒烟（年）	－0.045	0.371
年龄（岁）	0.084	0.272

续表

项目	相关系数 r/t	*P*
$PAaO_2$（mmHg）	- 0.317	0.009
PCO_2（mmHg）	0.206	0.068
FVC%pre	0.048	0.309
FEV1/FVC%	0.056	0.306
RV/TLC%	- 0.293	0.015
肺气肿积分（分）	- 0.412	0.001
肺纤维化积分(分）	- 0.191	0.081

3. 讨论

3.1 临床特征

本组 CPFE 综合征患者平均年龄 84 岁，目前文献[3, 5]报道的年龄 60 ~ 70 岁，本研究主要入组患者中高干病房病例占多数，故平均年龄较大。男性为主，38 例有吸烟史，且多数为大量吸烟者。动物实验证实[8]，香烟可趋化中性粒细胞在靶部位聚集，使弹性蛋白降解，出现肺气肿，并在修复过程中胶原和细胞外基质大量生成导致肺间质纤维化[9, 10]。卫小红[11]等研究显示：非特发性肺纤维化（IPF）患者纤维沉积明显，而 CPFE 综合征患者更偏重于炎性改变，提示 CPFE 综合征可能是一种特殊的病变而非 IPF 或慢性阻塞性肺疾病（COPD）两种疾病的简单相加。

CPFE 综合征患者临床症状以呼吸困难为主，并逐渐加重，本组患者 16.4% 有杵状指，78.2% 有下肺爆裂音，与目前报道一致[12]。

本研究 16 例以肺间质纤维化为首发疾病入院，39 例以肺气肿 /COPD 入院。季蓉等[4]报道的 11 例肺气肿合并肺间质纤维化的病例中 5 例以慢性支气管炎肺气肿为首发疾病，6 例以肺间质纤维化为首发疾病。

2011 年 IPF 诊断和治疗共识指出多数 IPF 患者存在胃食管反流，反复微量吸入是 IPF 的高危因素之一[13]。本研究发现 10 例经胃镜证实的反流性食管炎，CPFE 综合征与胃食管反流的关系有待大量的临床资料予以证实。

3.2 肺功能

肺功能有显著特点：肺容积相对正常，而弥散能力显著下降。尽管本研究入组患者的胸部 HRCT 上均有明确的肺气肿，但只有 28 例 $FEV_1/FVC < 70\%$。TLC 占预计值百分比

（105.43 ± 27.91）%，DLCO 占预计值百分比（72.54 ± 27.66）%，与目前报道的一致[14，15]。这是由于肺气肿所致的过度充气与纤维化所致的肺容积下降互相抵消，而两者对弥散能力的影响相互叠加所致。故肺容积不宜作为病情评价指标，门诊如果未查弥散功能，可能会导致漏诊[15]。

DLCO 占预计值百分比与吸烟量（$r = -0.324, P = 0.016$）及肺气肿积分（$r = -0.412, P = 0.002$）显著负相关，而与肺纤维化积分不相关。提示吸烟严重影响患者肺脏换气功能，而肺气肿对弥散功能下降起到更重要的作用。

3.3 影像学特点

HRCT 表现为双上肺间隔旁肺气肿或小叶中央型肺气肿，肺外周和下肺野为主的小叶间隔增厚、网状影、蜂窝影及牵拉性支气管扩张[3，11]。本组研究中肺气肿以小叶中心型为主，肺大泡 15 例，间隔旁肺气肿 11 例，肺纤维化以网格影表现为主（47 例）。间隔旁肺气肿可能是 CPFE 综合征独有的影像学特点，而吸烟相关肺气肿的典型表现是小叶中心性肺气肿。Akagi 等[16]的研究显示 CPFE 综合征患者 HRCT 上小叶中性肺气肿为主的占 41%，间隔旁肺气肿为主的占 54.2%。目前研究[17]一致认为 CPFE 综合征患者肺纤维化的分布和特征与 IPF 患者无明显差别。Cottin 等[3]的研究对 HRCT 所示肺气肿和纤维化病变缺少量化标准，本研究显示 55 例患者平均 EVS 评分（2.86 ± 2.86）分，平均肺纤维化积分（2.31 ± 1.56）分，肺气肿积分与 DLCO 下降显著相关（$r = -0.412$，$P = 0.002$）提示肺气肿和肺纤维化所占比例与肺功能相关。如影像学以肺气肿或纤维化占优势，相应的肺容积改变也倾向于正常或降低，治疗和预后也应符合其主要病变[18]。

3.4 病理及预后

单兆运等[19]报道了 30 例肺气肿患者经纤维支气管镜肺活检显示在肺气肿后期，肺间质纤维化改变逐渐取代了肺气肿的固有变化。杜敏捷等[20]对 41 例 COPD 并肺心病尸检病例进行分析，认为肺间质纤维化是病变随病程向肺组织深处发展的结果，可能是对炎症的一种修复反应。

本研究死亡患者中 7 例进行了尸体解剖，尸检显示肺上叶病理表现均为小叶中心型肺气肿和肺大泡，肺下叶病理主要表现为机化性肺炎（6 例），仅 1 例普通型间质性肺炎（UIP）。而目前有限的 CPFE 综合征患者的外科肺活检和尸体解剖病理显示，肺下叶的病理主要表现为普通型间质肺炎，有的病理表现无法分类[21]。关于 CPFE 综合征病理方面有待进一步研究。

CPFE 综合征患者有较高的肺动脉高压发生率[22，23]。本研究 16 例患者存在肺动脉高压，其中 9 例轻度，6 例中度，平均肺动脉压（59.31 ± 11.79）mmHg。Cottin 等[3]报道 61 例 CPFE 综合征患者有 47% 在诊断时合并肺动脉高压，心脏超声测量的肺动脉收缩压水平为

（48 ± 19）mmHg；在随诊中 55% 患者发生肺动脉高压。Grubstein 等 [21] 报道在 8 例重度吸烟的 CPFE 综合征患者中，7 例合并肺动脉高压。肺动脉压与预后密切相关（相对危险度为 4.03，95%CI 为 1.17～27.92，P = 0.03），1 年生存率仅为 60%，约 18% 的患者发生右心衰。本研究 16 例肺动脉高压患者中 4 例发生右心衰。

18 例患者出现 I 型呼吸衰竭。血气分析的显著特点为低氧血症，而二氧化碳升高不明显，$PA\text{-}aO_2$ 升高明显，并且 $PA\text{-}aO_2$ 与 DLCO 显著负相关（r = − 0.317，P = 0.018），说明肺气肿及肺纤维化导致 CPFE 综合征患者肺部受到双重损害，其换气功能严重受损。

7 例患者从 HRCT 上表现出病情进展，肺间质纤维化进展 2 例，肺气肿 / 肺大泡进展 3 例，1 例患者同时存在肺气肿和肺间质纤维化的进展。12 例患者在诊断 CPFE 综合征后出现肺癌，从诊断到发生肺癌的时间 2 个月～8 年，平均（3.56 ± 2.99）年。肺癌病理类型 5 例鳞癌，3 例腺癌，1 例小细胞肺癌，3 例未明确病理类型（PET-CT 提示肺癌）。且肿瘤标志物尤其是提示肺癌方面的多有升高（26 例 CEA 升高，18 例 SCC 升高，5 例 NSE 升高，18 例 CYFRA 升高）。Usui K 等 [18] 将 1143 例肺癌患者根据 HRCT 分为正常、肺气肿、肺纤维化、CPFE 综合征 4 组，发现 CPFE 综合征、肺气肿、肺纤维化合并肺癌分别有 101 例（8.9%），404 例（35.3%）和 15 例（1.3%），说明 CPFE 综合征患者较易合并肺癌。

CPFE 综合征患者易合并下呼吸道感染，本研究中因“肺炎，感染中毒性休克”死亡患者 13 例，故在治疗中应该时刻注意感染方面相关指标。

综上所述，吸烟是 CPFE 综合征发病的重要因素；呼吸困难为主要症状，血气分析出现明显低氧血症；易合并肺动脉高压，出现肺癌的几率升高；肺功能可提供早期诊断线索：弥散功能显著下降，肺容积可能会出现假正常化；影像学的肺气肿和肺纤维化所占比例与肺功能相关，HRCT 与肺功能指标相结合可以更好地评估病情。而其发病机制，病因等有待进一步研究。

参考文献

[1] Nakata H, KimotoT, Nakayama, et al. Diffuse peripheral lung disease: evaluation by high resolution Computed tomography [J]. Radiology 1985, 157(2): 181-185.

[2] Wiggins J, Steickland B, Turner WM. Combined crytogenic fibrosing alveolitis and emphysema: the value of high resolution computed tomography in assessment [J]. Respir Medicine, 1990, 84(5): 365-369.

[3] Cottin V, Nunes H, Brillet PY, et al. Combined pulmonary fibrosis and emphysema: a distinct under-recognised entity [J]. Eur Respir J, 2005, 26(4): 586-593.

[4] 季蓉，何权瀛．肺气肿合并肺间质纤维化的临床研究 [J]．中华结核和呼吸杂志，1999, 22(11): 666-668.

[5] 彭敏，蔡丰，田欣伦，等．肺纤维化合并肺气肿综合征八例并文献复习 [J]．中华结核和呼吸杂志，2010, 33(7): 515-518.

[6] Takasugi JE, Godwin JD. Radiology of chronic obstruct ion pulmonary disease [J]. Radio Clin Nor Am, 1998, 36(1): 29-55.

[7] Kazerooni E, Martinez F, Flint A. Thin-section CT obtained at 10-mm increments versus limited three level thin-section CT for idiopathic pulmonary fibrosis: correlation with pathologic scoring [J]. AJR Am J Roentgenol, 1997, 169(4): 977-983.

[8] Cisneros-Lira J, Gaxiola M, Ramos C, et al. Cigarette smoke exposure potentiates bleomycin-induced lung fibrosis in guinea pigs [J]. Am J Physicl Lung Cell Mol Physic1, 2003, 285(4): 949-956.

[9] Antoniou KM, Hansell DM, Rubens MB, et al. Idiopathic pulmonary fibrosis: outcome in relation to smoking status [J]. Am J Respir Crit Care Med, 2008, 177(2): 190-194.

[10] Nobukuni S, Watanabe K, Inoue J, et al. Cigarette smoke inhibits the growth of lung fibroblasts from patients with pulmonary emphysema[J]. Respirology, 2002, 7(3): 217-223.

[11] 卫小红，吴小燕，王军辉，等. 淋巴细胞和Ⅲ型前胶原氨基端肽与肺气肿合并肺纤维化的关系 [J]. 细胞与分子免疫学杂志，2010, 26(7): 675-678.

[12] Kitaguchi Y, Fujimoto K, Hanaoka M, et al. Clinical characteristics of combined pulmonary fibrosis and emphysema[J]. Respirology, 2010, 15(2): 265-271.

[13] Raghu G, Collard HR, Egan JJ, et al. An official ATS/ERS/JRS/ALAT statement: idiopathic pulmonary fibrosis: evidence-based guidelines for diagnosis and management[J]. Am J Respir Crit Care Med, 2011, 183(6): 788-824.

[14] Jankowich MD, Polsky M, Klein M, et al. Heterogeneity in combined pulmonary fibrosis and emphysema [J]. Respiration, 2008, 75(4): 111-117.

[15] Kurashima K, Takayanagi N, Tsuchiya N, et al. The effect of emphysema on lung function and survival in patients with idiopathic pulmonary fibrosis[J]. Respiratory, 2010, 15(5): 843-848.

[16] Akagi T, Matsumoto T, Harada T, et al. Coexistent emphysema delays the decrease of vitaI capacity in idiopathic pulmonary fibrosis[J]. Respir Med, 2009, 103(8): 1209-1215.

[17] Rogliani P, Mura M, Mattia P. HRCT and histopathological evaluation of fibrosis and tissue destruction in IPF associated with pulmonary emphysema[J]. Respiratory Medicine, 2008, 102(12): 1753-1761.

[18] Aduen JF, Zisman DA, Mobin SI, et al. Retrospective study of pulmonary function tests in patients presenting with isolated reduction in single-breath diffusion capacity: implications for the diagnosis of combined obstructive and restrictive lung disease [J]. Mayo Clin Proc, 2007, 82(1): 48-54.

[19] 单兆运，陈治安，马文富，等. 慢性阻塞性肺疾病的光镜、电镜及免疫病理研究 [J]. 中华结核和呼吸杂志，1990, 13(5): 311-313.

[20] 杜敏捷，王辰，曹大德，等. 慢性阻塞性肺疾病合并肺间质纤维化的病理学研究 [J]. 中华结核和呼吸杂志，1999, 22(1): 30-32.

[21] Grubstein A, Bendayan D, Schactman I, et al. Concomitant upper-lobe bullous emphysema, lower-lobe interstitial

fibrosis and pulmonary hypertension in heavy smokers: report of eight cases and review of the literature [J]. Respir Med, 2005, 99(8): 948-951.

[22] Nadrous HF, Pellikka PA, Krowka MJ, et al. Pulmonary hypertension in patients with idiopathic pulmonary fibrosis[J]. Chest, 2005, 128(4): 2393-2399.

[23] Mejía M, Carrillo G, Rojas-Serrano J, et al. Idiopathic pulmonary fibrosis and emphysema: decreased survival associated with severe pulmonary arterial hypertension [J]. Chest, 2009, 136(1): 10-15.

Factors Related to Ventricular Size and Valvular Regurgitation in Healthy Tibetans in Lhasa △

YANG Ying[1], CHEN Yundai[1], FENG Bin[1], JI Zhaxiduo[2], MAO Wei[3], ZHI Guang[1]

1. Department of Cardiology, Chinese PLA General Hospital, Beijing 100853, China
2. Department of Ultrasound Diagnosis, Tibet Second People's Hospital, Lhasa, Tibet 850000, China
3. Department of Internal Medicine, People's Hospital of Doilungdeqen County, Lhasa, Tibet 850000, China

Corresponding author: Dr. Guang Zhi, Department of Cardiology, Chinese PLA General Hospital, Beijing 100853, China. E-Mail: 13910994856@163. com

Abstract **Background** Lhasa is the main residence of Tibetans and one of the highest cities in the world. Its unique geography and ethnic population provide the chance to investigate the interactions among high altitude, ethnicity, and cardiac adaptation. Meanwhile, echocardiographic data about healthy Tibetans on a large scale are not available. This study aimed to analyze physiological factors related to ventricular size and valvular function in healthy Tibetans in Lhasa. **Methods** a representative sample of residents in Tibet was recruited using a multistage cluster random sampling method. Two-dimensional echocardiographic measurements and Doppler evaluation for valvular function were performed. Healthy Tibetans in Lhasa constituted the study population. Associations between physiological parameters and ventricular dimensions in healthy Tibetans were analyzed by canonical correlation analysis. Factors related to valvular regurgitations were determined by logistic regression analysis. **Results** The 454 healthy Tibetans (340 females and 114 male) in Lhasa were included in the final analysis. Canonical correlation analysis revealed that weight was positively correlated with the proximal right ventricular outflow diameter and the basal left ventricular linear dimension in both genders. Weight and pulse were negatively related to mild tricuspid regurgitation. Age was a positive factor for pulmonary and aortic regurgitations. The same was found between systolic blood pressure and mitral regurgitation. **Conclusions** Weight

△ 本文发表于：Chinese Medical Journal, 2017, 130 (19): 2316-2320.

is associated with ventricular size and valvular regurgitation. It should be of more concern in research of high altitude.

Key words Altitude; Echocardiography; Healthy Tibetans; Ventricular Regurgitation; Ventricular Size

1. Introduction

Lhasa is the administrative capital of the Tibet Autonomous Region of China. It is the main residence of Tibetans and has a population of 527, 300 [1]. Lhasa is also one of the highest cities in the world, at an altitude of 3 650 m. Compared to other parts of China, it is unique in ethnicity and geography.

Echocardiography is currently widely used in clinical practice for determination of cardiac size and function. Studies designed to analyze the interaction of high altitude and the heart by echocardiography have increased in Tibet. However, the target population for the identification of the prevalence of congenital heart diseases is frequently children and juveniles, and the information about adults is rare [2, 3]. Some studies have been carried out in hospitals for specific diseases, such as pulmonary hypertension, but they did not adequately represent the real world [4]. To the best of our knowledge, echocardiographic data about healthy Tibetans on a large scale are not available. An epidemiological study was carried out in Tibet for 3 years to identify the prevalence of chronic cardiac and pulmonary diseases. The study in Lhasa was the first to be completed. It provided the chance to analyze factors related to ventricular size and valvular function in healthy Tibetans.

2. Methods

2.1 Ethical approval

The study was conducted in accordance with the Declaration of Helsinki and was approved by the Local Ethics Committee of Fuwai Hospital. Informed written consent was obtained from all participants prior to their enrollment in this study.

2.2 Study population

This study was a part of a cross-sectional study in Tibet to identify the prevalence of chronic cardiac and pulmonary diseases. To include a sample cohort that is representative of the general population, we used multistage, cluster randomization and sampling methods. First, districts and counties in Tibet were divided into urban and rural areas. Two districts and four counties were drawn by the probability proportional to size method. Second, we selected two subdistricts from each district and two townships from each county using the simple random sampling (SRS) method. Third, we selected three communities from each subdistrict and three villages from each township by the SRS method. Finally, individuals aged 15 years or older, who have been living in the selected communities/villages for more than 0.6 years, were selected as candidates. It was estimated that the required sample size was approximately 1 000 in each district/county. The total number was divided into seven age groups (15 – 24 years, 25 – 34 years, 35 – 44 years, 45 – 54 years, 55 – 64 years, 65 – 74 years, and 75 years), and included an equal number of males and females. The number of participants in each age group was calculated from the percentage of population of the same age living in Tibet. Then, the number was divided among the six chosen communities/villages proportional to the number of candidates of this age. The final participants of each age group in a community/village were randomly chosen by SRS from the corresponding candidates.

Participants aged between 15 and 91 years were enrolled in the study. The data of basic information, physical examination, chest X-ray, electrocardiogram, echocardiography, and blood tests were collected from each participant.

Healthy Tibetans were recruited from the whole sample. The inclusion criteria required that participants should be aged 15 years or older, be of Tibetan ethnicity, and have normal results from the physical examination. The exclusion criteria were as follows: any self-reported and verified histories of coronary artery disease, structural heart disease, heart failure, stroke, endocrine diseases, acute or chronic respiratory diseases, anemia, connective tissue disease, or abnormal liver function. Participants with abnormal physical examinations and test results were also excluded, including hypertension (systolic blood pressure [SBP] ⩾ 140 mmHg, or diastolic blood pressure [DBP] ⩾ 90 mmHg or taking relevant drugs), obesity (body mass index [BMI] ⩾ 28.0 kg/m^2), hyperlipidemia (serum total cholesterol ⩾ 6.22 mmol/L, triglyceride ⩾ 2.26 mmol/L, or taking relevant drugs), diabetes mellitus (fasting blood glucose > 7.0 mmol/L or taking relevant drugs), abnormal renal function (serum creatinine ⩾ 110 μmol/L), abnormal electrocardiography (Q wave, arrhythmia, or bundle block), valvular stenosis (any degree), more than mild valvular regurgitation, wall motion abnormalities and pericardial effusion on echocardiographic recordings, Assessment Test Score of chronic obstructive pulmonary disease > 20, forced expiratory volume in 1 s/forced vital capacity ratio from pulmonary function test < 0.7, emphysema, pulmonary heart disease, pneumonia, bronchiectasis, tuberculosis, and pleural effusion on chest X-ray. Professional athletes, pregnant or lactating women, participants addicted to alcohol, and participants with inadequate echocardiographic images were excluded from the study.

2.3 Acquisition of echocardiographic information

Echocardiography was performed by two certified physicians using two Vivid-Q portable machines (Vingmed-Ultrasound General Electric, Horten, Norway). The two-dimensional (2D) images were acquired and measured in the parasternal (standard long-and short-axis images) and apical 4-chamber views, according to the guidelines of the American Society of Echocardiography (ASE) [5]. Right ventricular (RV) linear dimensions were estimated from an RV-focused apical 4-chamber view. The basal RV linear dimension (RVbd) was defined as the maximal transverse dimension in the basal one-third of the RV inflow at end diastole. The proximal RV outflow diameter (RVOTprox) was defined as the linear dimension measured from the anterior RV wall to the interventricular septal-aortic junction in the parasternal long-axis view at end diastole. The pulmonary artery (PA)dimension was measured between the valve and the bifurcation point at end diastole [6]. The basal left ventricular linear dimension (LVbd) was defined as the maximal transverse dimension in the basal one-third of the LV inflow at end diastole. M-mode was used to measure the diameters of the left ventricle at end diastole (LVEDD) and at end systole (LVESD). The cursor was perpendicular to the LV long axis and located at the level of the mitral valve leaflet tips. Electronic calipers were positioned at the interface between the myocardial wall and cavity. The assessment of valvular stenosis and regurgitation by Doppler was carried out as recommended by the ASE [7, 8]. LVEF was derived from M-mode using the Teichholz formula, except for the regional abnormality of wall motion. At least 3 cardiac cycles were recorded for each view, and the optimal view was selected for measurement.

2.4 Statistical analysis

Qualitative data were expressed as percentages (%). The normality distribution of continuous variables was assessed using the Kolmogorov – Smirnov test. Data with normal distribution were presented as the mean ± standard deviation and compared by independent sample t-test. Data with skewed distribution were presented as the median (Q1, Q3) and compared by the Wilcoxon rank-sum test. Comparison between skewed data and normal data was performed by the Wilcoxon rank-sum test. Associations between physiological parameters and ventricular dimensions were analyzed by canonical correlation analysis. Factors related to valvular regurgitation were analyzed using a multivariate unconditional logistic regression (method: forward: LR). Two-tailed $P < 0.05$ was considered statistically significant. Statistical analyses were performed using the SPSS software version 19.0 (IBM SPSS, Armonk, NY, USA).

3. Results

3.1 Demographic features and cardiac measurements

Individuals in the Chengguan district and Doilungdeqen county in Lhasa were recruited for the epidemiological study. The 894 participants (571 females and 323 males) from the Chengguan district and 570 participants (371 females and 199 males) from the Doilungdeqen county were initially screened. The 454 healthy Tibetans (340 females and 114 male) in Lhasa met the inclusion and exclusion criteria and were included in the final analysis. Demographic features of the study sample are summarized in Table 1. The study revealed that the values of height, weight, and blood pressure were higher in males than those of females (all $P < 0.01$), whereas no significant differences in age, pulse, and blood oxygen saturation (SpO_2) were found between males and females (all $P > 0.05$). The parameters of ventricular measurements (including RVbd, LVbd, LVEDD, and LVESD) were larger in males than those of females (all $P < 0.01$).

3.2 Factors related to ventricular size

In healthy Tibetans, the canonical correlation analysis method was used to analyze the relationship between physiological parameters (U1 = age, height, weight, pulse, SBP, DBP, and SpO_2) and right/left ventricular dimensions (Vr = PA, RVOTprox and RVbd/Vl = LVbd, LVEDD, and LVESD)in males and females. In these cases, the first (and the second) canonical correlation was statistically significant, as summarized in Tables 2 and 3. However, the second canonical correlations were usually omitted in conventional way because of their small coefficients compared to the first ones.

Table 1 Demographic features and cardiac measurements of healthy Tibetans in Lhasa (n = 454)

Items	Males (n = 114)	Females (n = 340)	Statistical values	P
Age (years)	44.0 (20.8, 57.0)	39.5 (30.0, 51.0)	− 0.70*	0.49
Height (cm)	165.4 ± 7.4	156.7 ± 5.5	− 10.50†	< 0.01
Weight (kg)	62.3 ± 8.8	56.4 ± 7.5	− 6.95†	< 0.01
Pulse (beat/min)	76.0 (68.8, 87.3)	77.0 (70.0, 85.0)	− 0.48*	0.63
SBP (mmHg)	122.0 (114.0, 130.0)	119.0 (110.0, 127.0)	− 3.13*	< 0.01
DBP (mmHg)	75.0 (69.0, 83.0)	73.0 (67.0, 80.0)	− 2.62*	< 0.01
SpO_2 (%)	88.0 (85.0, 91.3)	89.0 (85.0, 91.8)	− 0.86*	0.39
PA (mm)	18.0 (16.0, 19.0)	17.0 (16.0, 19.0)	− 0.49*	0.63

续表

Items	Males (n = 114)	Females (n = 340)	Statistical values	P
RVOTprox (mm)	25.0 (23.0, 26.3)	23.0 (21.0, 26.0)	– 3.38*	< 0.01
RVbd (mm)	29.3 ± 5.2	27.5 (25.0, 30.0)	– 3.87*	< 0.01
LVbd (mm)	41.0 (38.0, 45.0)	38.0 (36.0, 41.0)	– 5.97*	< 0.01
LVEDD (mm)	43.0 (40.0, 45.0)	39.0 (36.0, 42.0)	– 6.42*	< 0.01
LVESD (mm)	28.0 (26.0, 30.0)	26.0 (24.0, 28.0)	– 4.79*	< 0.01
TR, n (%)	22 (19.3)	57 (16.8)	—	—
PR, n (%)	2 (1.8)	7 (2.1)	—	—
MR, n (%)	2 (1.8)	4 (1.2)	—	—
AR, n (%)	4 (3.5)	5 (1.5)	—	—

Data are presented as median (Q1, Q3) for skewness distribution and mean ± SD for normal distribution. *Z values; †t values. SBP: Systolic blood pressure; DBP: Diastolic blood pressure; SpO_2: Blood oxygen saturation; PA: Pulmonary artery; RVOTprox: Proximal right ventricular outflow diameter; RVbd: Basal right ventricular linear dimension; LVbd: Basal left ventricular linear dimension; LVEDD: Left ventricular end-diastolic diameter; LVESD: Left ventricular end-systolic diameter; SD: Standard deviation; TR: Tricuspid regurgitation; PR: Pulmonary regurgitation; MR: Mitral regurgitation; AR: Aortic regurgitation.

Table 2 Canonical correlation coefficients and hypothesis testing between physiological parameters and right ventricular dimensions in healthy Tibetans

Canonical correlation	Males					Females				
	Coefficients	Wilk's	χ^2	df	P	Coefficients	Wilk's	χ^2	df	P
First	0.46	0.73	56.14	21.00	< 0.01	0.40	0.82	78.57	21.00	< 0.01
Second	0.22	0.87	25.69	12.00	0.01	0.16	0.97	12.99	12.00	0.37
Third	0.14	0.95	9.05	5.00	0.11	0.09	0.99	3.15	5.00	0.68

Table 3 Canonical correlation coefficients and hypothesis testing between physiological parameters and left ventricular dimensions in healthy Tibetans

Canonical correlation	Males					Females				
	Coefficients	Wilk's	χ^2	df	P	Coefficients	Wilk's	χ^2	df	P
First	0.53	0.68	70.45	21.00	< 0.01	0.34	0.83	73.27	21.00	< 0.01
Second	0.20	0.93	13.21	12.00	0.35	0.15	0.94	24.78	12.00	0.02
Third	0.18	0.97	5.84	5.00	0.32	0.11	0.98	9.92	5.00	0.08

According to the calculation of standardized canonical coefficients, the first canonical relationship between U1 and Vr can be presented as the following equations:

$U1 = -0.57\ age + 0.32\ height - 0.56\ weight + 0.14\ pulse - 0.25\ SBP + 0.02\ DBP + 0.28\ SpO_2$,

$Vr = 0.11PA - 1.07\ RVOTprox + 0.32\ RVbd$ for men; and

$U1 = -0.29\ age - 0.09\ height - 0.77\ weight + 0.23\ pulse - 0.12\ SBP + 0.03\ DBP + 0.14\ SpO_2$,

$Vr = -0.47\ PA - 0.60\ RVOTprox - 0.35\ RVbd$ for women.

The first canonical relationship between U1 and Vl can be presented as the following equations:

$U1 = 0.23\ age - 0.07\ height - 0.59\ weight + 0.76\ pulse + 0.08\ SBP - 0.16\ SBP - 0.04\ SpO_2$,

$Vl = -0.59\ LVbd - 0.47\ LVEDD - 0.10\ LVESD$ for men; and

$U1 = -0.29\ age + 0.04\ height + 0.72\ weight - 0.27\ pulse + 0.54\ SBP - 0.25\ DBP - 0.01\ SpO_2$,

$Vl = 0.83\ LVbd + 0.15\ LVEDD + 0.15\ LVESD$ for women.

In those equations, larger standardized canonical coefficients indicated a closer relationship between physiological parameters and ventricular sizes. Parameter and dimension with the same tokens (both are plus signs or minus signs)exhibited a positive relationship with each other. Similarly, opposite tokens represented an inverse relationship. Canonical correlation analysis revealed that weight was positively correlated with RVOTprox for the right ventricle and LVbd for the left ventricle in both genders. In addition, age was positively correlated with RVOTprox and pulse was negatively correlated with LVbd in men. SBP was positively correlated with LVbd in women.

3.3 Factors related to valvular regurgitations

Participants with valvular stenosis (any degree) and more than mild valvular regurgitation were excluded from the study population. The unconditional logistic regression model was used to evaluate whether gender, age, height, weight, pulse, SBP, DBP, or SpO_2 were related to mild valvular regurgitation. Table 4 summarizes the independent factors for mild valvular regurgitation. Weight and pulse were negatively related to mild tricuspid regurgitation (TR). Age was a positive factor for pulmonary regurgitation (PR)and aortic regurgitation (AR). The same was found for SBP and mitral regurgitation (MR).

Table 4 Factors related to mild valvular regurgitation calculated by logistic regression

Valvular regurgitation	Factors	β	*P*	EXP (β)	95%CI
Mild TR	Weight (kg)	− 0.05	< 0.01	0.95	0.92 − 0.98
	Pulse (beat/min)	− 0.03	0.02	0.97	0.95 − 0.99

续表

Valvular regurgitation	Factors	β	*P*	EXP (β)	95%CI
Mild PR	Age (years)	0.04	0.03	1.04	1.00 – 1.09
Mild MR	SBP (mmHg)	0.06	0.04	1.06	1.00 – 1.12
Mild AR	Age (years)	0.09	< 0.01	1.10	1.05 – 1.14

TR: tricuspid regurgitation; PR: pulmonary regurgitation; MR: mitral regurgitation; AR: aortic regurgitation; SBP: systolic blood pressure; CI: confidential interval.

4. Discussion

The effect of age on cardiac size has been long studied. Recently, a nationwide, population-based study of healthy Han Chinese adults revealed that values of RV anterior wall thickness and RV anteroposterior dimension gradually increase with age in both genders, while values of the RV outflow tract, RV middle dimension, and RV basal dimension did not vary with age in either gender. [9] The article partly supports the results of our study. In our study, the RVOTprox is measured in the same view as that used to acquire the RV anteroposterior dimension. Therefore, their changes are positively correlated with age. In addition, the RVbd does not vary with age in both genders. The aforementioned study also revealed that there were no significant differences in the LV outflow tract among the six age groups in both genders. This result is similar with the little relationship between age and the LV dimensions in our study. Age is a risk factor for PR and AR. A study of autopsy specimens of normal hearts concludes that, in both genders, all indexed mean valve circumferences progressively increased throughout adult life, and this trend was greater for the semilunar valves than for the atrioventricular valves [10]. Additionally, aortic root dilatation is one of most common causes of AR [11]. A study assessing clinical determinants of valvular regurgitation from the Framingham Heart Study revealed that the clinical determinants of MR were age, hypertension, and BMI. The determinants of AR were age and male gender [12]. The relationship between blood pressure and MR might enhance at high altitude though SBP is in normal range.

Weight is neglected in most studies. In fact, the study of autopsy specimens of normal hearts reported that body weight was a better predictor of normal heart weight than body surface area or height, and its mean values per decade was significantly increased in women [10]. High altitude presents a hypoxic environment that adversely affects human physiology and metabolism. A study reported that body weight decreased following exposure to high altitude [13]. Tibetan women give birth to larger babies than Han Chinese women, which is one of the physiological adaptations to high altitude-related hypoxia [14]. It is postulated that weight might be one of the indicators of adaptation, development, and nourishment at high altitudes. Therefore, it is positively related to cardiac size.

Hypoxia at high altitudes causes pulmonary vasoconstriction, which improves the matching of perfusion to alveolar ventilation. On the other hand, hypoxic vasoconstriction induces pulmonary hypertension and increases RV afterload [15]. TR is related to pulmonary hypertension and RV enlargement at high altitudes [16]. However, it was found that SpO_2 is not related to mild TR in our study. It is the weight negative for TR. This means that mid TR at high altitudes might be related to physiological development rather than hypoxia.

The limitations of the current study included the following: only 2D measurements were reported in the present study, short of Doppler data and volumes of chambers. In the future, more advanced and accurate echocardiographic technologies will be applied in Tibet and produce more valuable information for high altitudes.

In conclusion, weight is associated with ventricular size and valvular regurgitation. It should be of more concern in research of high altitude.

5. Financial support and sponsorship

The study was supported by a grant from Healthcare Scientific Research in the Public Interest of the China National Health and Family Planning Commission (No.201402002).

6. Conflicts of interest

There are no conflicts of interest.

References

[1] Annual by Selected Cities. NBS: National Bureau of Statistics of China; 2014. Available from: http: //www. data. stats. gov. cn/English/easyquery. htm?cn = E0105. [Last accessed on 2016 Aug 20].

[2] Hou HJ, Liu WX, Meng RY, Qin J, Su JL, Jing RF, et al. Prevalence of Congenital Heart Diseases of Rural Tibetan Pupils in Suo Country in Naqu Area. The National Echocardiographic Academic Conference (in Chinese). Beijing: Chinese Association of Ultrasound in Medicine and Engineering; 2014. p.234-5.

[3] Wang J, Wang ZN, Li SZ, Wang LJ, Chen ZD, Wang HY, et al. An investigation of congenital heart diseases of 6500 pupils in Lhasa (in Chinese). Tibet Sci Technol 2002; 1: 12-4. doi: 10.3969/j. issn.1004-3403.2002.01.005.

[4] Li JM, Cen WJ. The value of pulse Doppler for estimating pulmonary hypertension in highland (in Chinese). Tibet Med 1991; 3: 5-7.

[5] Lang RM, Badano LP, Mor-Avi V, Afilalo J, Armstrong A, Ernande L, et al. Recommendations for cardiac chamber

quantification by echocardiography in adults: An update from the American Society of Echocardiography and the European Association of Cardiovascular Imaging. J Am Soc Echocardiogr 2015; 28: 1-39. e14. doi: 10.1016/j. echo.2014.10.003.

[6] Rudski LG, Lai WW, Afilalo J, Hua L, Handschumacher MD, Chandrasekaran K, et al. Guidelines for the echocardiographic assessment of the right heart in adults: A report from the American Society of Echocardiography endorsed by the European Association of Echocardiography, a registered branch of the European Society of Cardiology, and the Canadian Society of Echocardiography. J Am Soc Echocardiogr 2010; 23: 685-713. doi: 10.1016/j. echo.2010.05.010.

[7] Zoghbi WA, Enriquez-Sarano M, Foster E, Grayburn PA, Kraft CD, Levine RA, et al. Recommendations for evaluation of the severity of native valvular regurgitation with two-dimensional and Doppler echocardiography. J Am Soc Echocardiogr 2003; 16: 777-802. doi: 10.1016/S0894-7317(03)00335-3.

[8] Baumgartner H, Hung J, Bermejo J, Chambers JB, Evangelista A, Griffin BP, et al. Echocardiographic assessment of valve stenosis: EAE/ASE recommendations for clinical practice. J Am Soc Echocardiogr 2009; 22: 1-23. doi: 10.1016/j. echo.2008.11.029.

[9] Yao GH, Deng Y, Liu Y, Xu MJ, Zhang C, Deng YB, et al. Echocardiographic measurements in normal Chinese adults focusing on cardiac chambers and great arteries: A prospective, nationwide, and multicenter study. J Am Soc Echocardiogr 2015; 28: 570-9. doi: 10.1016/j. echo.2015.01.022.

[10] Kitzman DW, Scholz DG, Hagen PT, Ilstrup DM, Edwards WD. Age-related changes in normal human hearts during the first 10 decades of life. Part II (Maturity): A quantitative anatomic study of 765 specimens from subjects 20 to 99 years old. Mayo Clin Proc 1988; 63: 137-46. doi: 10.1016/S0025-6196(12)64946-5.

[11] Olson LJ, Subramanian R, Edwards WD. Surgical pathology of pure aortic insufficiency: A study of 225 cases. Mayo Clin Proc 1984; 59: 835-41. doi: 10.1016/S0025-6196(12)65618-3.

[12] Singh JP, Evans JC, Levy D, Larson MG, Freed LA, Fuller DL, et al. Prevalence and clinical determinants of mitral, tricuspid, and aortic regurgitation (the Framingham Heart Study) Am J Cardiol 1999; 83: 897-902. doi: 10.1016/S0002-9149(98)01064-9.

[13] Chen KT, Chen YY, Wu HJ, Chang CK, Lee WT, Lu YY, et al. Decreased anaerobic performance and hormone adaptation after expedition to Peak Lenin. Chin Med J (Engl) 2008; 121: 2229-33.

[14] Bigham AW. Genetics of human origin and evolution: High-altitude adaptations. Curr Opin Genet Dev 2016; 41: 8-13. doi: 10.1016/j. gde.2016.06.018.

[15] Naeije R, Dedobbeleer C. Pulmonary hypertension and the right ventricle in hypoxia. Exp Physiol 2013; 98: 1247-56. doi: 10.1113/expphysiol.2012.069112.

[16] Po JR, Meeran T, Davey R, Benza R, Raina A. Tricuspid regurgitation is associated with pulmonary hemodynamics and right ventricular dysfunction in pulmonary arterial hypertension but does not alter the geometry of right ventricular contraction. J Am Coll Cardiol 2016; 67: 2056. doi: 10.1016/S0735-1097(16)32057-5.

不同地区民族心脏形态及功能的对比分析△

杨　瑛，智　光，朱庆磊，周姗姗，王增武，陈　蒙，陈韵岱，冯　斌

解放军总医院心内科　北京 100853

通讯作者：冯斌，E-mail：1694063952@qq.com

摘　要　目的　以超声心动图测量为手段，就西藏地区藏族健康人群与北京地区汉族健康人群进行比较，研究高原环境、不同民族心脏形态、功能的交互作用。**方法**　以西藏地区常住人口为总体，采用分层4阶段随机抽样方法抽取调查对象，筛选高原藏汉健康人群，与平原汉族健康人群心脏测量数据进行比较。**结果**　通过高原藏族健康人群与平原汉族健康人群匹配后心脏功能比较，发现高原藏族右心室测量指标要大于平原汉族人群；而大血管测量指标主动脉窦内径、升主动脉内径、主肺动脉内径，部分左心测量指标包括左房左右径、前后径、左室舒张末内径、左室射血分数方面，高原藏族要小于平原汉族。主肺动脉、升主动脉、三尖瓣环收缩期位移汉族健康人群高于藏族健康人群，其余指标两组之间差异无显著性。**结论**　高原环境与右心室扩大、左心室受抑制有关。民族因素对高原适应人群心脏影响有限。

关键词　高原；藏族；超声心动图

Comparison of cardiac measurements on echocardiography in different region and enthnicity

Ynag Ying, Zhi Guang, Zhu Qinglei, Zhou Shanshan, Wang Zengwu, Chen Meng, Chen Yundai, Feng Bin

Department of Cardiology, Chinese PLA General Hospital, Beijing 100853

Corres ponding author: Feng Bin, Email: 1694063952@qq.com

Abstract　Objective　The goal of the manuscript is to present the impact of difference region and ethnicity on echocardiographic measurements. **Methods**　A representative sample of residents in Tibet was recruited using

△　本文发表于：中华保健医学杂志，2017，19（6）：471-473.

a multistage cluster random sampling method. Healthy Tibetans and healthy Han highlanders were drawn from the sample. We explored discrepancy of cardiac chamber diameters and function in healthy Han lowlanders versus healthy Tibetans, and Healthy Han highlanders versus Tibetans. **Results:** Healthy Tibetans had higher measurements of right ventricle, less diameters of aortic artery, pulmonary artery, left atrium and left ventricle in diastolic end, and lower left ventricular ejection fraction than healthy Han lowlanders after matching. Whereas, healthy Tibetans had similar cardiac chamber diameters and function with healthy Han highlanders, except main pulmonary artery, ascending aortic artery and tricuspid annular plane systolic excursion. **Conclusions** There is apparent difference in cardiac structure between Han lowlanders and Tibetans, little difference between healthy Han highlanders and Tibetans.

Key words High altitude; Tibetan; Echocardiograph

西藏自治区地处我国西南边陲，平均海拔在 4 000 m 以上，是藏族人群主要聚集地，具有地理和民族上的特殊性。北京地处华北平原北部，是我国政治经济中心，具有平原地区和汉族人群的代表性。两地区健康人群心脏超声测量数据库的建立，为评价地区、民族差异对心脏形态及功能的影响提供了依据。

1. 对象与方法

1.1 对象

1.1.1 高原健康人群 以西藏地区常住人口为总体，采用分层 4 阶段随机抽样方法抽取调查对象。首先在西藏自治区内按城乡分为 2 层，每层内采用与容量大小成比例的概率抽取所需数量的区 / 县，然后在被抽中的区 / 县中采用简单随机抽样（simple random sampling，SRS）方法抽取两个街道 / 乡镇，再在被抽中的街道 / 乡镇中采用 SRS 法抽取 3 个居 / 村委会后，在被抽中的居 / 村委会中采用 SRS 方法随机抽取调查个体。该调查纳入西藏地区 4 688 人，同时收集调查对象个人信息、病史；行体格检查、心电图、胸片及超声心动图检查；血尿化验等资料。

排除标准:（1）冠状动脉疾病、先天性心脏病、心力衰竭、心电图异常（病理性 Q 波、心律失常及完全性束支阻滞），超声心动图发现瓣膜狭窄（任何程度），瓣膜反流（中到重度，三尖瓣反流速度 > 2.8 m/s），室壁运动障碍、心包积液;（2）中风、高血压、高脂血症（血清总胆固醇 > 6.22 mmol/L 或三酰甘油 > 2.26 mmol/L，或正在服用调脂药物）、糖尿病、肥胖（体质量指数 > 28.0 kg/m^2）;（3）急性或慢性呼吸道疾病病史、慢性阻塞性肺疾病评估测试评分 > 20，经胸片检查，排除肺气肿、肺心病、肺炎、支气管扩张、结核、胸腔积液，肺功能检查支气管扩张剂吸入后的 1 秒率约 0.7；（4）贫血、肝脏疾病，肾功能异常（血清

肌酐 > 110 μmol/L），酒精成瘾者；（5）职业运动员，怀孕或哺乳期妇女；（6）图像质量差不能分析。

高原藏族健康人群纳入标准：年龄 > 15 岁，藏族，体格检查正常。

高原汉族健康人群纳入标准：年龄 > 15 岁，汉族，体格检查正常。

研究最终获得健康藏族人群 1 820 人，其中男性 707 人，女性 1 113 人；林芝地区 286 人，拉萨地区 694 人，那曲地区 575 人，日喀则地区 265 人。高原汉族健康人群 224 人，其中男性 128 人，女性 96 人；林芝地区 40 人，拉萨地区 91 人，那曲地区 18 人，日喀则地区 75 人。

1.1.2　平原汉族健康人群　2006 年阜外医院联合解放军总医院报告北京地区健康人群心脏测量参考值范围，入选健康汉族成年人 2 332 例，其中男性 1 133 人，女性 1 199 人[1]。所有受试者排除高血压、冠心病、糖尿病等慢性病史，体格检查正常。

1.2　方法

参照《中国成年人超声心动图检查测量指南》，比较两个数据库人群的心脏测量指标，包括主动脉窦、升主动脉、主肺动脉等，左心室射血分数的计算（LVEF）采用 Simpson 双平面法[2]。

采用倾向评分匹配的统计学方法，在高原藏族健康人群与平原汉族健康人群之间匹配年龄、身高、体重、性别、脉搏基本人体测量指标，卡钳值设为 0.000 1，重新建立以上指标均衡的比较组，对心脏测量指标比较。在藏汉两组之间建立基本人体测量指标均衡的比较组，增加血氧饱和度，卡钳值设为 0.000 05。

1.3　统计学处理

应用 SPSS 24.0 软件统计分析，正态分布连续变量以 $\bar{x}$ + SD 表示，偏态分布连续变量以中位数（四分位数）表示，分类变量表述为数量。偏态资料两组间、偏态资料与正态资料比较采用秩和检验，分类变量两组间比较采用卡方检验或连续校正法或 Fisher 确切概率法。以双侧 $P < 0.05$ 为差异有统计学意义。

2. 结果

2.1　高原藏族健康人群与平原汉族健康人群心脏形态与功能比较

两地区原始数据库基本人体测量指标比较差异明显，经匹配后获得 439 对新样本，性别、年龄、身高、体重、脉搏指标得到均衡，见表 1。

表 1　匹配后高原藏族健康人群与平原汉族健康人群人体测量指标比较

组别	例数	性别（男/女）	年龄（岁）	身高（cm）	体重（kg）	脉搏（次/分）
高原藏族	439	200/239	41（33, 51）	163.7（159.0, 170.0）	62.0 ± 8.5	72（65, 78）
平原汉族	439	191/248	40（28, 51）	163.0（158.0, 170.0）	62.0（55.0, 70.0）	72（66, 79）
P 值		0.54	0.10	0.80	0.88	0.43

匹配后，两组间右房左右径、左室横径、左室收缩末前后径差异无显著性（P＞0.05）。右室测量指标，包括右室横径、右室前后径、右室壁厚度，高原藏族要大于平原汉族人群；其他大血管测量指标包括主动脉窦内径、升主动脉内径、主肺动脉内径，部分左心测量指标，包括左房左右径、前后径、左室舒张末内径、LVEF，高原藏族要小于平原汉族人群，差异均有统计学意义（P＜0.05，表 2）。

表 2　高原藏族与平原汉族心脏测量指标比较 [mm，P_{50}（P_{25}，P_{75}），$\bar{x} \pm s$]

组别	例数	主动脉窦	升主动脉	主肺动脉	右室横径	右室前后径	右室壁厚度	右房左右径
高原藏族	439	26（25, 29）	26（23, 28）	18（17, 20）	30（26, 35）	23（21, 25）	5（4, 5）	32（29, 35）
平原汉族	439	28.5（26.5, 31）	27（25, 30）	20.7 ± 2.7	28.9 ± 4.4	21.7（19.3, 24.6）	4（3.5, 4.7）	31.3 ± 4.7
P 值		0.00	0.00	0.00	0.00	0.00	0.00	0.24

组别	左房左右径	左房前后径	左室横径	左室舒张末期前后径	室间隔舒张末厚度	左室收缩末前后径	LVEF（%）
高原藏族	31（28, 33）	27（25, 30）	41（38, 43）	42（39, 45）	9（8, 9）	28（26, 31）	64（58, 68）
平原汉族	34.1 ± 4.8	30.5 ± 4.0	41.3（37.8, 44.3）	46.3 ± 4.1	8.4（7.4, 9.4）	28.7（26, 31.2）	64.6 ± 7.7
P 值	0.00	0.00	0.06	0.00	0.00	0.05	0.01

注：LVEF. 左心室射血分数。

2.2　高原藏族健康人群与高原汉族健康人群心脏形态与功能比较

高原藏族健康人群与高原汉族健康人群经匹配后得到新样本 72 对，各项指标得到均衡，其中主肺动脉、升主动脉、三尖瓣环收缩期位移（TAPSE）3 项指标汉族健康人群高于藏族健康人群，且差异有统计学意义（P＜0.05，表 3、表 4）；其余指标无差异。

表 3　匹配后高原藏族健康人群与高原汉族健康人群人体测量指标比较（$\bar{x} \pm s$）

组别	例数	性别（男 / 女）	年龄（岁）	身高（cm）	体重（kg）	脉搏（次 /min）	血氧饱和度（%）
高原藏族	72	36/36	32.3 ± 12.7	161.3 ± 8.0	59.1 ± 9.8	74.6 ± 11.1	89.2 ± 4.9
高原汉族	72	28/44	35.5（26.5, 39）	160.4 ± 9.5	57.1 ± 9.5	77（71, 82）	90.0（87.3, 93.0）
P 值		0.18	0.17	0.56	0.22	0.11	0.32

表 4　高原藏族与高原汉族心脏测量指标比较 [mm，P_{50}（P_{25}，P_{75}），$\bar{x} \pm s$]

组别	例数	主动脉窦	升主动脉	主肺动脉	右室横径	右室前后径
高原藏族	72	25.2 ± 3.2	24.2 ± 3.7	18.4 ± 2.5	28.5（25.3, 33.8）	22.5（20, 25）
高原汉族	72	26（23, 29）	27（22, 29）	20（19, 22）	30（27, 32）	22（20, 24）
P 值		0.06	0.01	0.02	0.48	0.20

组别	右室壁厚度	右房左右径	左房左右径	左房前后径	左室横径
高原藏族	5（4, 5）	30.9 ± 4.1	30（28, 33）	27（24, 29）	40（38, 42）
高原汉族	5（4, 5）	30（27, 32.8）	31（29, 33）	26.9 ± 3.6	39（36, 41）
P 值	0.27	0.35	0.38	0.58	0.05

组别	左室舒张末期前后径	室间隔舒张末厚度	左室收缩末前后径	LVEF（%）	TAPSE
高原藏族	42（39, 44.8）	9（8.0, 9.0）	27.4 ± 4.2	65.3 ± 5.8	23（20, 26）
高原汉族	42（39, 43.8）	9（8, 9）	28.7 ± 4.4	67（63, 70）	25（21, 27.8）
P 值	0.63	0.11	0.09	0.41	0.03

注：TAPSE. 三尖瓣环收缩期位移。

3. 讨论

健康人群暴露于低氧环境，首先出现与低氧血症相对应的心率加快、心输出量增加，几天之后人群逐步适应，心率仍然加快，但每搏量下降，心输出量恢复到既往水平[3-4]。但有研究认为健康人群进入高原后减小的是左心形态，而不是 LVEF[5]。高原常驻健康人群中也可观察到左心受缺氧影响而发生改变，较平原前往高原适应人群，前者 LVEF 较低[6]。既往有研究通过二维斑点追踪技术对平原迁往高原适应人群（平原、高原两个状态）、高原常驻健康人群及患有高原病人群 4 种人群的心脏进行了比较，发现高原常驻健康人群较平原人群 LVEF 差异没有显著性，但心指数、每搏量、左室舒张 / 收缩容量、组织多普勒二尖瓣环 S 波 /E 波均低于平原人群，提示低氧环境对左心形态及功能有不同程度的抑制[7]。本研究结果与既往研究提示的左心抑制状态相符。

关于高原低氧环境对右心的影响，有文献指出，无论是患者还是健康人群，进入高原后均会出现右心扩大、TAPSE 降低[8]。既往一项尸检曾明确提出高原儿童较平原地区存在右心室肥厚[9]。我国曾有一项研究对平原、高原常驻健康儿童进行了超声心动图对比检查，发现高原地区儿童平均肺动脉压较高，右心室扩张，出生 14 年后右心室相对肥厚，左、右心室的收缩和舒张功能降低[10]。以上研究提示在高原缺氧环境中，右心扩大，右心室肥厚是适应性改变。

但本研究测量指标差异可能缘于藏、汉民族差异。有研究通过 DNA 分析，藏族与蒙古人、东亚人具有较近的亲缘关系[11]。高原健康儿童研究也提示右心大小、厚度与功能在高原藏汉儿童之间无明显差异[10]。本研究结果同样验证了民族因素在心脏形态及功能上的影响较小。

本研究通过对不同地区民族健康人群心脏测量数据比较，高原环境与右室扩大，左心受抑有关，民族因素对心脏形态与功能影响有限。 需要注意的是，本研究由于数据库不同，或存在观察者间、超声机器间偏倚。

参考文献

[1] 喻丽华，杨浣宜，智光，等．北京地区 2 332 例中正常人二维超声心动图测量系列正常值及其影响因素 [C]．合肥：全国超声医学学术会议 .2006.

[2] 中华医学会超声医学分会超声心动图学组．中国成年人超声心动图检查测量指南 [J]．中华超声影像学杂志，2016，25（8）：645-666.

[3] Naeije R, Melot C, Mols P, et al. Effects of vasodilators on hypoxic pulmonary vasoconstriction in normal man [J]. Chest, 1982, 82(4): 404-410.

[4] Klausen K. Cardiac output in man in rest and work during and after acclimatization to 3,800 m [J]. J Appl Physiol, 1966, 21(2): 609-616.

[5] Fowles RE, Hultgren HN. Left ventricular function at high altitude examined by systolic time intervals and M-mode echocardiography [J]. Am J Cardiol, 1983, 52(7): 862-866.

[6] Huez S, Faoro V, Guenard H, et al. Echocardiographic and tissue Doppler imaging of cardiac adaptation to high altitude in native highlanders versus acclimatized lowlanders [J]. Am J Cardiol, 2009, 103(11): 1605-1609.

[7] Dedobbeleer C，Hadefi A，Pichon A，et al. Left ventricular adaptation to high altitude: speckle tracking echocardiography in lowlanders, healthy highlanders and highlanders with chronic mountain sickness [J]. Int J Cardiovasc Imaging, 2015, 31(4): 743-752.

[8] de Vries ST, Kleijn SA, van't Hof AW, et al. Impact of high altitude on echocardiographically determined cardiac morphology and function in patients with coronary artery disease and healthy controls [J]. Eur J Echocardiogr,

2010, 11(5): 446-450.

[9] Arias-Stella J, Recavarrea S. Right Ventricular hypertrophy in native children living at high altitude [J]. Am J Pathol, 1962, 41(1): 55-64.

[10] 齐海英，徐素雅，马如雁，等．中国高原地区与平原地区儿童心脏解剖和功能以及肺循环血液动力学的比较咱 J 暂．中华心血管病杂志，2015，43（9）：774-781.

[11] 温有锋．西藏藏族起源初探 [D]．中国医科大学，2007.

西藏地区正常藏族人群心脏形态及瓣膜关闭不全相关因素分析△

杨　瑛[1]，冯　斌[1]*，智　光[1]，朱庆磊[1]，周珊珊[1]，陈　蒙[1]，王增武[2]，陈韵岱[1]

1. 中国人民解放军总医院心内科；2. 国家心血管病中心社区防治部中国医学科院阜外医院
通讯作者：陈韵岱，Email: cyundai@vip. 163. com;
*，共同第一个作者：王增武，Email: wangzengwu@foxmail. com

摘　要　目的　探讨高原环境下正常藏族人群心脏形态及瓣膜关闭不全的相关因素。**方法**　以西藏地区常住人口为总体，采用分层四阶段随机抽样方法抽取调查对象，在所有调查人群中筛选正常藏族人群。收集调查对象的个人信息、病史、行体格检查、实验室（血尿）检查、心电图、X 线胸片及超声心动图检查，包括径线测量及瓣膜功能评价。采用典型相关及逻辑回归的方法分析正常藏族人群心脏结构、瓣膜功能相关因素。**结果**　西藏地区共 4 688 人参加调查，获得正常藏族人群共计 1 820 人，其中拉萨地区 694 人、那曲地区 575 人、林芝地区 286 人、日喀则地区 265 人。典型相关分析发现，正常藏族人群右心室测量主要相关生理学指标为年龄、血氧饱和度、体重，男女差异不大；左心室测量主要相关生理学指标为：体重、年龄、身高，同样性别差异较小。通过回归分析发现，体重、脉搏、血氧饱和度是轻度三尖瓣关闭不全的负相关因素；年龄是轻度二尖瓣、主动脉瓣关闭不全的正相关因素（P 均 < 0.01）。**结论**　在高原地区藏族人群中，年龄、体重是心脏形态、瓣膜轻度关闭不全相关因素，在心脏疾病分析中应重视其作用。

关键词　高原；心脏瓣膜疾病；超声心动描记术；藏族

Correlation Factor Analysis for Cardiac Morphology and Valvular Regurgitation in Normal Tibetan Population at High Altitude Area

Yang Ying, Feng Bin, Zhi Guang, Zhu Qinglei, Zhou Shanshan, Chen Meng, Wang Zengwu, Chen

△　本文发表于：中国循环杂志，2018，33（2）：172-177.

Yundai.
Department of Cardiology, PLA General Hospital, Beijing (100853), China
Corresponding Author: CHEN Yun-dai, Email: cyundai@vip.163.com; WANG Zeng-wu, Email:wangzengwu@foxmail.com

Abstract Objective To explore the correlation factors for cardiac morphology and valvular regurgitation in normal Tibetan population at high altitude area. **Methods:** Based on Tibetan permanent resident population, a 4-stage cluster random sampling was conducted to drawn normal Tibetan subjects. Personal information and medical history were collected; physical parameters including blood and urine tests, ECG, chest X-ray and echocardiography were examined; cardiac morphology and valvular stenosis and regurgitation were detected. Canonical correlation study and Logistic regression analysis were performed to investigate the correlation factors for cardiac structure and function. **Results:** A population of 4 688 in Tibetan area were involved and 1 820 normal subjects were studied including 694 from Lhasa, 575 from Naqu, 286 from Nyingchi and 265 from Shigatse area. Canonical correlation analysis revealed that in normal Tibetan population, the major relevant physiological parameters for measuring right ventricle were age, blood oxygen saturation and body weight; for left ventricle were body weight, age and height; gender had no real differences. Logistic regression analysis presented that body weight, pulse and blood oxygen saturation were negatively related to mild tricuspid regurgitation; age was positively related to mild mitral and aortic regurgitations, all $P < 0.01$. **Conclusions** Age and body weight were the correlation factors for cardiac morphology and mild valvular regurgitation in normal Tibetan population at high altitude area, which should be alert in heart disease investigation.

Key words High altitude; Heart valve disease; Echocardiography; Tibetan

西藏自治区地处我国西南边陲，平均海拔在 4 000 m 以上，是藏族人群主要聚集地。受多因素影响，该地区人群心脏形态及瓣膜功能相关研究处于相对空白状态。2014 年，解放军总医院心血管内科与西藏自治区医学专业人员密切合作，历时 3 年，在该地区开展慢性心肺疾病流行病学调查，获得大量数据，为研究正常藏族人群心脏形态与瓣膜功能提供了依据。

1. 资料与方法

1.1 调查对象

本研究以西藏地区常住人口为总体，采用分层四阶段随机抽样方法抽取调查对象，详见图 1。以 2007 年西藏地区的高血压患病率作为估计值 [1]，结合冠心病、慢性阻塞性肺疾病、脑卒中患病率的样本需求，考虑实施难度，计划在西藏抽取 15 岁以上人群 6 000 人进行调查，每个区 / 县分配 1 000 人。以年龄 / 性别分层，每层数量按照各年龄阶段占西藏总人口的百分比计算，经调整不应答率、男女各半获得。

1.2 调查方法

收集调查对象个人信息、病史；所有调查对象行体格检查、实验室（血尿）检查、心电图、X 线胸片及超声心动图检查。超声图像采集：采用 Vivid-I 机型，M3S 探头。由两名有资质医师采集。常规探查各切面、测量心脏各腔室大小、室壁厚度、及左、右心室功能；评价各组瓣膜形态及活动度，有无狭窄及关闭不全。径线测量及瓣膜功能评价按美国超声协会推荐的标准[2-4]。

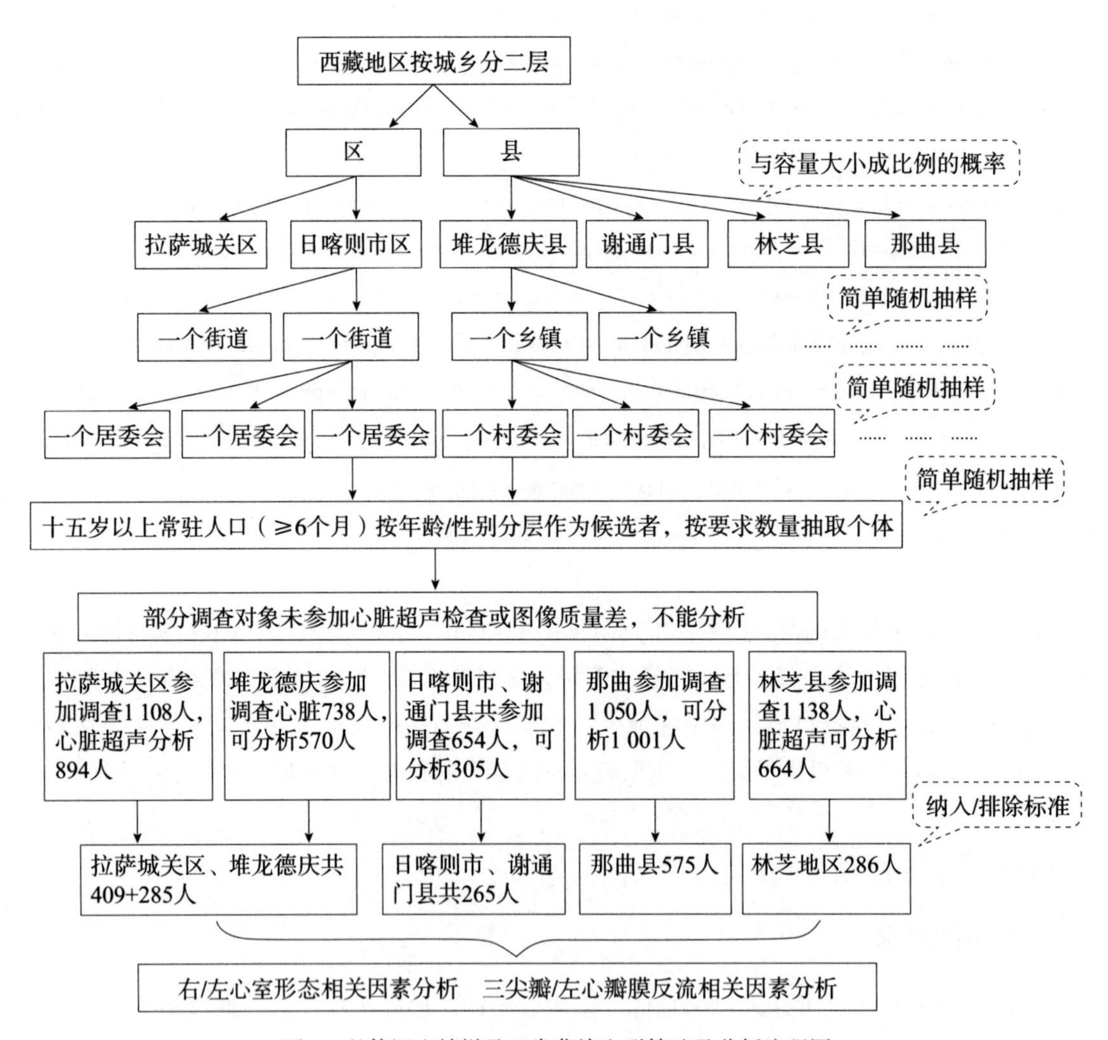

图 1　整体调查抽样及正常藏族人群筛选及分析流程图

入选标准：在所有调查人群中筛选正常藏族人群，符合以下标准：年龄在 15 岁以上，藏族，体格检查正常。

排除标准：冠状动脉疾病、先天性心脏病、心力衰竭、高血压、卒中、高脂血症（血清总胆固醇≥ 6.22 mmol/L 或甘油三酯≥ 2.26 mmol/L，或正在服用调脂药物）、糖尿病、急性或慢性呼吸道疾病病史、慢性阻塞性肺疾病评估测试评分 < 20 分、贫血、肝脏疾病、肾功能异常（血清肌酐≥ 110 μmol/L）、肥胖（体重指数≥ 28.0 kg/m^2）、心电图异常（病理性 Q 波、心律失常及完全性束支阻滞）、超声心动图检查发现任何程度瓣膜狭窄、瓣膜关闭不全（中－重度、三尖瓣反流速度> 2.8 m/s）、室壁运动障碍、心包积液。

经 X 线胸片检查，排除肺气肿、肺原性心脏病、肺炎、支气管扩张、结核、胸腔积液。肺功能检查支气管扩张剂吸入后的 1 秒率 < 0.7。图像质量差不能分析需排除。

1.3 统计学方法

所有统计分析应用 SPSS 24.0 统计软件进行。（1）分类变量以数量或百分比表示，正态分布连续变量以均数 ± 标准差表示，偏态分布连续变量以中位数（四分位数）表示。偏态资料两组间或与正态资料两组间相比较采用秩和检验。（2）正常藏族人群心脏形态相关因素分析，采用典型相关方法。按性别分别建立基本生理指标（SET1）：年龄、身高、体重、脉搏、血氧饱和度与心脏测量指标（SET2）：右心室：主肺动脉宽度、右心室前后径、右心室横径；左心室：左心室横径、左心室舒张末期前后径、左心室收缩末期前后径，一对间接典型相关变量（见下公式）。（3）瓣膜关闭不全相关因素分析：以性别、年龄、身高、体重、脉搏、血氧饱和度为自变量，以三尖瓣、二尖瓣、主动脉瓣关闭不全为应变量，建立逻辑回归方程。双侧 $P < 0.05$ 为差异有统计学意义。

2. 结果

2.1 总体基本情况

整体西藏地区共 4 688 人参加调查，获得正常藏族人群共 1 820 人，其中拉萨地区 694 人、那曲地区 575 人、林芝地区 286 人、日喀则地区 265 人。正常藏族人群基本生理学指标及心脏测量指标见表 1。表 1 提示瓣膜关闭不全中轻度三尖瓣关闭不全的检出率最高；男女之间年龄、血氧饱和度无差异，女性脉搏比男性快，而男性心脏测量指标均大于女性，差异均有统计学意义（P 均 < 0.05）。

表 1　正常藏族人群基本生理学及心脏测量指标［中位数（四分位数）］

指　　标	男（$n=707$）	女（$n=1\ 113$）	总体（$n=1\ 820$）
年龄（岁）	36（26, 47）	38（28, 48）	37（27, 47）
身高（cm）	166（162, 170.5）	156.9（153, 160）*	160（155, 165）
体重（kg，$\bar{x} \pm s$）	62.1 ± 9.6	55.3（49.6, 61.3）*	58.0 ± 9.2
脉搏（次 /min）	73（66, 81）	74（68, 82）*	74（67, 81）
血氧饱和度（%）	89（85, 92）	89（85, 92）	89（85, 92）
主肺动脉宽度（mm）	18（17, 20）	18（16, 19）*	—
右心室前后径（mm）	23（21, 25）	22（20, 24）*	—
右心室横径（mm）	30（26, 33）	28（24, 32）*	—
左心室横径（mm）	41（39, 44）	39（36, 41）*	—
左心室舒张末期前后径（mm）	43（41, 46）	40（37, 43）*	—
左心室收缩末期前后径（mm）	28（26, 31）	26（24, 29）*	—
轻度三尖瓣关闭不全[例（%）]	—	—	238（13.1）
轻度二尖瓣关闭不全[例（%）]	—	—	49（2.7）
轻度主动脉瓣关闭不全[例（%）]	—	—	25（1.4）

注：与男性比较 *$P<0.05$.　—：未计算。

2.2　正常藏族人群心室形态相关因素分析

正常藏族男性右心室典型相关系数及假设检验结果（表 2）：正常藏族男性右心室三个典型相关系数，经假设检验可以发现第一、第二对典型相关变量之间相关性可以成立，第三对相关性不成立。基本生理学指标与右心室测量指标之间的关系转化为第一、第二对典型相关变量之间的关系。

表 2　正常藏族男性右心室典型相关系数及假设检验结果（$n=707$）

	典型相关系数	Wilk's	Chi-SQ	DF	P 值
1	0.565	0.620	335.731	15.000	0.000
2	0.289	0.910	66.459	8.000	0.000
3	0.086	0.993	5.264	3.000	0.153

根据标准化典型变量系数，第一对典型变量函数为：

$$\begin{cases} SET1 = -0.607\text{年龄} - 0.357\text{身高} - 0.195\text{体重} + 0.079\text{脉搏} - 0.493\text{血氧饱和度} \\ SET2 = -0.805\text{主肺动脉} - 0.304\text{右心室横径} - 0.085\text{右心室前后径} \end{cases}$$

第二对典型变量函数为：

$$\begin{cases} SET1 = 0.286\text{年龄} - 0.344\text{身高} + 0.710\text{体重} + 0.106\text{脉搏} - 0.706\text{血氧饱和度} \\ SET2 = 0.246\text{主肺动脉} - 0.769\text{右心室横径} + 0.795\text{右心室前后径} \end{cases}$$

在第一对典型变量中，基本生理学指标中年龄的系数较大，而心脏测量中主肺动脉系数最大，结合回归系数符号相同，可以认为年龄与主肺动脉宽度呈正相关。而第二对典型变量中，生理学指标中体重、血氧饱和度系数较大，右心室测量在右心室横径、右心室前后径上的系数较大。这说明体重与右心室前后径呈正相关，与右心室横径呈负相关；血氧饱和度与右心室横径呈正相关，与右心室前后径呈负相关。

正常藏族女性右心室典型相关系数及假设检验结果（表3）：正常藏族女性右心室三个典型相关系数，三对典型相关变量之间的相关性可以成立，但第三对典型变量相关系数非常小，可以忽略不计。

表3　正常藏族女性右心室典型相关系数及假设检验结果（*n* = 1 113）

	典型相关系数	Wilk's	Chi-SQ	DF	*P*值
1	0.517	0.687	416.538	15.000	0.000
2	0.238	0.937	72.224	8.000	0.000
3	0.084	0.993	7.897	3.000	0.048

根据标准化典型变量系数，第一对典型变量函数为：

$$\begin{cases} SET1 = -0.566\text{年龄} - 0.252\text{身高} - 0.277\text{体重} + 0.095\text{脉搏} - 0.518\text{血氧饱和度} \\ SET2 = -0.549\text{主肺动脉} - 0.553\text{右心室横径} - 0.150\text{右心室前后径} \end{cases}$$

第二对典型变量函数为：

$$\begin{cases} SET1 = 0.223\text{年龄} - 0.183\text{身高} + 0.661\text{体重} - 0.119\text{脉搏} - 0.721\text{血氧饱和度} \\ SET2 = 0.067\text{主肺动脉} - 0.478\text{右心室横径} + 0.957\text{右心室前后径} \end{cases}$$

在第一对典型变量中，基本生理学指标中年龄和血氧饱和度系数较大，而右心室测量中主肺动脉、右心室横径系数较大，结合回归系数符号相同，认为年龄、血氧饱和度与主肺动脉、右心室横径呈正相关。第二对典型变量中，基本生理学指标主要受体重和血氧饱和度影响，右心室测量在右心室前后径系数较大。体重与右心室前后径呈正相关，血氧饱和度与右心室前后径呈负相关。

正常藏族男性左心室典型相关系数及假设检验结果（表4）：正常藏族男性左心室三个典型相关系数，经假设检验可以发现第一、第二对典型相关变量之间相关性可以成立，第三对相关性不成立。基本生理学指标与左心室测量指标之间的关系转化为第一、第二对典型相关变量之间的关系。

表 4　正常藏族男性左心室典型相关系数及假设检验结果（*n* = 707）

	典型相关系数	Wilk's	Chi-SQ	DF	Sig.
1	0.406	0.786	168.565	15.000	0.000
2	0.239	0.942	42.069	8.000	0.000
3	0.036	0.999	0.901	3.000	0.825

根据标准化典型变量系数，第一对典型变量函数为：

SET1 = − 0.030 年龄 − 0.134 身高 − 0.725 体重 + 0.503 脉搏 − 0.085 血氧饱和度
SET2 = − 0.384 左心室横径 − 0.439 左心室舒张末期前后径 − 0.376 左心室收缩末期前后径

第二对典型变量函数为：

SET1 = 0.737 年龄 + 0.732 身高 − 0.760 体重 + 0.219 脉搏 + 0.555 血氧饱和度
SET2 = − 0.043 左心室横径 − 1.104 左心室舒张末期前后径 + 1.287 左心室收缩末期前后径

在第一对典型变量中，基本生理学指标中体重系数较大，而左心室测量中左心室舒张末期前后径系数较大，结合回归系数符号相同，可以认为体重与左心室舒张末期前后径呈正相关。而第二对典型变量中，生理学指标中年龄、身高、体重系数均较大，左心室测量在左心室舒张末期前后径、左心室收缩末期前后径上的系数较大。这说明年龄大、身材高的正常藏族男性左心室收缩末期前后径大；体重大的正常藏族男性左心室舒张末期前后径大。

正常藏族女性左心室典型相关系数及假设检验结果（表 5）：显示正常藏族女性左心室的三个典型相关系数，经假设检验可以看到第一、第二对典型相关变量之间相关性可以成立，而第三对典型变量相关不成立。

表 5　正常藏族女性左心室典型相关系数及假设检验结果（*n* = 1 113）

	典型相关系数	Wilk's	Chi-SQ	DF	*P* 值
1	0.363	0.848	181.958	15.000	0.000
2	0.128	0.978	25.147	8.000	0.001
3	0.078	0.994	6.735	3.000	0.081

根据标准化典型变量系数，第一对典型变量函数为：

$$\begin{cases}\text{SET1} = -0.345\text{年龄} - 0.232\text{身高} - 0.589\text{体重} + 0.320\text{脉搏} - 0.246\text{血氧饱和度}\\ \text{SET2} = -0.482\text{左心室横径} - 0.348\text{左心室舒张末期前后径} - 0.382\text{左心室收缩末期前后径}\end{cases}$$

第二对典型变量函数为：

$$\begin{cases}\text{SET1} = -0.764\text{年龄} - 0.588\text{身高} + 0.860\text{体重} - 0.195\text{脉搏} - 0.309\text{血氧饱和度}\\ \text{SET2} = 0.131\text{左心室横径} + 1.160\text{左心室舒张末期前后径} - 1.385\text{左心室收缩末期前后径}\end{cases}$$

在第一对典型变量中，生理学指标中体重的系数最大，而左心室测量中左心室横径系数较大，结合回归系数符号相同，认为体重与左心室横径呈正相关。第二对典型变量中，生理指标主要受年龄、身高、体重影响，左心室测量在左心室舒张末期前后径、左心室收缩末期前后径上的系数较大。体重与左心室舒张末期前后径呈正相关，年龄、身高与左心室收缩末期前后径呈正相关。

经以上典型相关分析，可以发现正常藏族人群右心室测量主要相关生理学指标为年龄、血氧饱和度、体重，男女差异不大；左心室测量主要相关生理学指标为：体重、年龄、身高，同样性别差异较小。

2.3 心脏瓣膜关闭不全相关因素分析

因健康人群入选时排除了瓣膜病，应变量为无、轻度瓣膜关闭不全。以性别、年龄、身高、体重、脉搏、血氧饱和度为自变量建立逻辑二分类回归方程。结果如表 6 所示。体重、脉搏、血氧饱和度为三尖瓣轻度关闭不全的负相关因素。年龄为二尖瓣、主动脉瓣轻度关闭不全的正相关因素。

表 6 正常藏族人群轻度瓣膜关闭不全相关因素分析

因　素	β	*P* 值	EXP（β）	95%CI
三尖瓣轻度反流				
体重（kg）	−0.046	0.000	0.955	0.94 ~ 0.97
脉搏（次 / 分）	−0.019	0.003	0.981	0.969 ~ 0.994
血氧饱和度（%）	−0.048	0.000	0.953	0.929 ~ 0.977
轻度二尖瓣关闭不全				
年龄（岁）	0.032	0.002	1.032	1.012 ~ 1.053
轻度主动脉瓣关闭不全				
年龄（岁）	0.075	0.000	1.077	1.047 ~ 1.109

3. 讨论

所谓“正常人”不是指机体任何器官、组织的形态和机能正常的人，而是排除了影响所研究指标的疾病和有关因素的同质人群[5]。本研究借鉴心脏超声研究中关于“正常人群”的定义，对“正常”进行界定[6]。

关于年龄对心脏形态及功能影响，一项全国范围内正常汉族人群超声心动图测量结果[6]提示主肺动脉宽度随年龄增加而增加。同时该研究指出在无论性别差异，左心室舒张末期内径随年龄增长轻度减低；男性人群中左心室收缩末期内径随年龄增长减低，而女性中则不变。本研究结果显示无论性别，年龄与主肺动脉呈正相关，这一点即使存在低氧的环境差异，与正常汉族人群是相符合的。在正常藏族人群中左心室舒张末期前后径与年龄呈负相关，但属于次要相关。本研究结果提示左心室收缩末期内径与年龄呈正相关，这一点与以上研究不符，不能排除与地区民族差异有关，需要进一步研究。另一方面，年龄是左心瓣膜关闭不全的正相关因素。研究发现，随着年龄的增大，瓣环周长在不断增大，这一点在主动脉瓣、肺动脉瓣上表现尤为突出[7]。而主动脉瓣环扩张及升主动脉扩张是导致主动脉瓣关闭不全的主要原因[8]。Framingham 研究认为主动脉瓣关闭不全相关因素包括年龄、男性；二尖瓣关闭不全相关因素包括年龄、高血压、体重指数[9]。所以即使存在低氧高原环境，左心瓣膜关闭不全情况符合一般流行病学规律。

体重因素在研究中往往被忽略。事实上，针对健康心脏解剖分析发现[7]，体重是心脏重量良好预测指标，在一定程度上代表了心脏的生长发育状态。而且在高原低氧对机体作用中，机体内水、脂肪的代谢会发生改变，从而引起体重明显下降[10]。有研究总结在安第斯山区及藏族人群中出生时体重增加是对高原环境的适应性改变之一[11]。推测在高原特殊环境下，体重是机体适应能力的一个指标，代表机体生长发育营养状态。所以，体重与左、右心室形态均相关，并与三尖瓣轻度关闭不全呈负相关。

高原低氧环境会引起肺血管收缩以达到通气灌注匹配的目的，但这种适应性反应的另一面是肺动脉高压[12]。在高原环境中，低氧导致肺动脉压增高、肺血管阻力增加、右心扩大，并最终导致三尖瓣关闭不全[13]。所以血氧饱和度与右心室形态密切相关。但右心室本身形态不规则，虽然本研究采用了通用的多角度测量以提高对右心室形态的概括能力，但仍存在右心室横径与右心室前后径受血氧饱和度影响而变化不一致的情况，提示右心室受低血氧影响而发生的形态改变可能同样不规则，并非简单线性或平面变化，可能采用最新的右心室三维立体重建测量才能全面反映。本研究也发现高血氧饱和度是轻度三尖瓣关闭不全的负相关因素，这与既往观点认为轻度三尖瓣关闭不全为功能性改变相左，提示在高原环境中应重视轻度三尖瓣关闭不全的发生，并随访其发展变化。

参考文献

[1] 古桑拉姆，平措扎西，蔡玉霞，等. 西藏农牧区高血压患病率、知晓率、治疗率和控制率的调查 [J]. 中国医药指南，2010, 27(8): 79-81. DOI: 10. 3969/j. issn. 1671-8194. 2010. 27. 050.

[2] Lang RM, Badano LP, Moravi V, et al. Recommendations for cardiac chamber quantification by echocardiography in adults: an update from the American Society of Echocardiography and the European Association of Cardiovascular Imaging[J]. Eur Heart J Cardiovasc Imag, 2015, 16(3): 233-270. DOI: 10. 1093/ehjci/jev014.

[3] Zoghbi WA, Enriquez-Sarano M, Foster E, et al. Recommendations for evaluation of the severity of native valvular regurgitation with two-dimensional and Doppler echocardiography [J]. J Am Soc Echocardiogr, 2003, 16 (7): 777-802. DOI: 10. 1016/S0894-7317(03) 00335-3.

[4] Baumgartner H, Hung J, Bermejo J, et al. Echocardiographic assessment of valve stenosis: EAE/ASE recommendations for clinical practice [J]. J Am Soc Echocardiogr, 2009; 22 (1): 1-23. DOI: 10. 1016/j. echo.2008.11. 029.

[5] 田凤调. 医学正常值的统计研究方法 [M]. 北京：人民卫生出版社，1990.

[6] Yao GH, Deng Y, Liu Y, et al. Echocardiographic measurements in normal Chinese adults focusing on cardiac chambers and great arteries: a prospective, nationwide, and multicenter study[J]. J Am Soc Echocardiogr, 2015, 28(1): 570-579. DOI: 10. 1016/j. echo. 2015. 01.022.

[7] Kitzman DW, Scholz DG, Hagen PT, et al. Age-related changes in normal human hearts during the first 10 decades of life. Part II (Maturity): a quantitative anatomic study of 765 specimens from subjects 20 to 99 years old[J]. Mayo Clinic Proceedings, 1988, 63(2): 137-146. DOI: 10. 1016/S0025-6196(12)64946-5.

[8] Olson LJ, Subramanian R, Edwards WD. Surgical pathology of pure aortic insufficiency: a Study of 225 Gases[J]. Mayo Clinic Proceedings, 1985, 59(12): 835-841. DOI: 10. 1016/S0025-6196(12)65618-3.

[9] Singh JP, Evans JC, Levy D, et al. Prevalence and clinical determinants of mitral, tricuspid, and aortic regurgitation (the Framingham Heart Study)[J]. Am J Cardiol, 1999, 83(6): 897-902. DOI: 10. 1016/S0002-9149(98)01064-9.

[10] Vats P, Ray K, Majumadar D, et al. Changes in cardiovascular functions, lipid profile, and body composition at high altitude in two different ethnic groups[J]. High Alt Med Biol, 2013, 14(1): 45-52. DOI: 10. 1089/ham. 2012. 1071.

[11] Bigham AW. Genetics of human origin and evolution: high-altitude adaptations[J]. Curr Opin Genet Dev, 2016, 41(12): 8-13. DOI: 10.1016/j. gde. 2016. 06. 018.

[12] Naeije R, Dedobbeleer C. Pulmonary hypertension and the right ventricle in hypoxia[J]. Exp Physiol, 2013,

98(8): 1247-1256. DOI: 10.1113/expphysiol. 2012. 069112.

[13] Po JR, Meeran T, Davey R, et al. Tricuspid regurgitation is associated with pulmonary hemodynamics and right ventricular dysfunction in pulmonary arterial hypertension but does not alter the geometry of right ventricular contraction[J]. J Heart Lung Transpl, 2016, 35(4): S356-S356. DOI: 10.1016/j. healun. 2016. 01.1024.

2010～2015年我国新疆疾控机构传染病控制人力资源变化趋势分析△

刘 靓[1]，夏代提古丽·苏拉衣曼[2]，吴 静[3]

1. 中国疾病预防控制中心传染病预防控制所，北京 102206
2. 新疆维吾尔自治区疾病预防控制中心
3. 中国疾病预防控制中心，慢病社区处

通讯作者：吴静，E-mail：wujingcdc@163.com

摘 要 目的 了解2010～2015年我国新疆疾控机构传染病控制人力资源状况和变化趋势，为进一步优化疾控人员配置提供依据。**方法** 利用全国疾病预防控制基本信息网络直报系统收集人员信息，运用R软件分析疾控机构的人力资源数据。**结果** 2010～2015年全国疾控机构传染病防控人员数量总体呈上升趋势，传染病防控人员所占比例呈逐年增加的趋势。新疆疾控机构从事传染病控制的人员总数自2011年起逐年增加，且整体人员受教育程度逐年递增。从与全国的比较结果看，2012～2015年间新疆自治区级疾控中心传染病防控人员所占比例高于西部地区平均水平，但低于东、中部地区平均水平；而地市级疾控中心的比例高于东、中部地区平均水平，低于西部地区水平；新疆区县级疾控中心的传染病防控人员比例则高于东、中部和西部地区。**结论** 新疆疾控机构人员的数量和受教育程度自2011年起均有所提高；自治区级和区县级的相关人员配置均高于西部地区平均水平，建议增加地市级人员配置。此外，也建议新疆结合当地疾病谱的转变对人员整体结构进行适当调整。

关键词 疾控机构；新疆维吾尔自治区；传染病控制；人力资源

Analysis of Variation Trends of Human Resources in Charge of Communicable Disease Control in Centers for Disease Control and Prevention in Xinjiang from 2010 to 2015

Liu Jing[1], Xiadaitiguli Sulayiman[2], Wu Jing[3]

△ 本文发表于：中国现代医药杂志，2017，19（5）：14-19.

1 Institute for Communicable Disease Control and Prevention, 3. Department of Chronic Disease and Community-acquired Disease, Chinese Center for Disease Control and Prevention, Beijing 102206

2. Xinjiang Uygur Autonomous Region Center for Disease Control and Prevention

Abstract **Objective** To understand the distribution and variation trends of human resources in charge of communicable diseases control in Centers for Disease Control and Prevention (CDCs) in Xinjiang Uygur Autonomous Region in China during 2010 ~ 2015 and provide data support for optimizing allocation of manpower in local CDCs' human resource departments. **Methods** Used the Information System of China Disease Control and Prevent to analyse the distribution and variation trends of health workforce in CDCs with R software. **Results** The total number of the CDCs in China increased during 2010 ~ 2015, the percentage of the employees combating communicable diseases increased year by year. The number of employees in charge of communicable disease control increased year by year in Xinjiang and the education level of the professional employees in CDCs in Xinjiang Uygur Autonomous Region had been upgraded every year since 2011. During the period of 2012 ~ 2015, the proportions of working against communicable diseases in provincial CDCs in Xinjiang were lower than that in eastern and middle China, and higher than that in western China, while in municipal level, proportions were larger than that in eastern and middle China and smaller than that in western China, in county level, the proportions in Xinjiang were the greatest compared with eastern, middle and western China. **Conclusions** The numbers and education level of health workforce in CDCs in Xinjiang have increased since the year 2011. In both provincial and county levels, the situation in terms of human resources relating to disease control were more preferable than that in western China, and for CDCs in municipal and county level, more employees should be hired. It is also suggested that the departments in charge of communicable disease control in CDCs in Xinjiang, corresponding to the population increases in the local area due to the population mobility, could recruit more health professionals.

Key words Center for Disease control institutions; Xinjiang Uygur Autonomous Region; Infectious disease control; Human resources; Trends

近年来，新发和再发传染病对我国公民的健康影响依然严重，特别是在新疆地区，近年来传染病仍有暴发的趋势[1, 2]，因此有必要对当地疾控机构传染病相关人员的现状和变化趋势进行分析。本研究从区域、层级和时间等维度分析我国不同级别和地区的疾控中心中负责传染病防控工作的人员数量。再将新疆维吾尔自治区的疾控中心人员进行单独分析，并将其与全国总体数据进行对比，以了解当地传染病控制人员分配情况，并为当地疾控中心人员配置方案的优化给出建议。

1. 材料与方法

1.1 一般资料

全部数据来自 2010 ~ 2015 年全国疾病预防控制基本信息统计分析系统。该系统接收全国所有省、地市和区县级疾控中心的上报信息，并且由经过省级疾控中心统一培训的人员承担填报工作，每年的人员信息填报率高于 93%。数据信息经过严格的核查，其准确率比较高。

1.2 统计学方法

使用 Excel 2011 进行数据录入，之后用 R 软件对数据进行逻辑核对后，分不同地区、不同年份以及不同层级，对疾控中心机构及人员数量进行统计学描述和趋势分析。

表 1　2010 ~ 2015 年各疾控机构数与传染病控制人员数及其所占比例 [*n*（%）]

级别	2010 年		2011 年		2012 年	
	机构数	传染病控制人员数	机构数	传染病控制人员数	机构数	传染病控制人员数
省级	32	932（7.62）	31	820（7.07）	34	875（7.31）
地市级	353	2 691（7.29）	342	2 913（7.56）	352	2 894（7.38）
区县级	2 948	12 009（9.04）	2 899	13 379（9.15）	2 940	13 944（9.26）
合计	3 333	15 632（8.59）	3 272	17 112（8.72）	3 326	17 713（8.78）

级别	2013 年		2014 年		2015 年	
	机构数	传染病控制人员数	机构数	传染病控制人员数	机构数	传染病控制人员数
省级	32	861（7.24）	32	865（7.49）	32	888（7.38）
地市级	347	3 021（7.56）	347	3 010（7.54）	348	3 045（7.61）
区县级	2 972	14 494（9.28）	2 974	14 482（9.30）	2 966	15 012（9.37）
合计	3 351	18 376（8.83）	3 353	18 357（8.86）	3 346	18 945（8.92）

2. 结果

2.1 全国基本情况

2010 年全国在统计信息系统内登记的疾控中心数量共 3 333 个。这个数量在 2011 年有所减少，在 2013 ~ 2014 年间有所增加，分别为 3 351 和 3 353 个；随后在 2015 年减少至

3 346 个。全国疾控中心传染病防控人员总数仅在 2014 年略有减少，其他年份总体呈增长趋势；在 2014 年人数略有减少，为 18 357 人。但是传染病防控人员所占比例，在本研究关注的 6 年间，从 2010 年的 8.59% 到 2015 年的 8.92%，呈逐年增高的趋势，见表 1。

2.2 全国不同级别疾控机构传染病控制人员情况

从 2010～2015 年，负责传染病控制的人员在省级疾控中心的所占比例在 2010 年达到最高为 7.62%，在 2011 年降至 6 年来最低为 7.07%。而地市级疾控中心人数和构成比则在 2012 年和 2014 年出现小幅减少；6 年间，从事传染病控制的人员人数构成比在 7.29%～7.56% 之间波动。每年区县级疾控中心负责传染病控制的人员构成比例均高于省级和地市级，其比例最低约为 9.04%，最高约达到 9.37%，并且在 6 年间逐年增加，见表 1。

2.3 全国不同地区疾控中心传染病控制人员情况

总体看，东、中、西部地区均呈现上升的趋势。2010～2015 年，每年东部地区的传染病控制人员人数均少于西部和中部地区；6 年间，西部和东部地区人数呈逐年增加的趋势，但中部地区在 2014 年出现了人员减少的情况，见图 1。每年，西部地区从事传染病控制的人员构成比例，均高于东部和中部地区，见表 2。

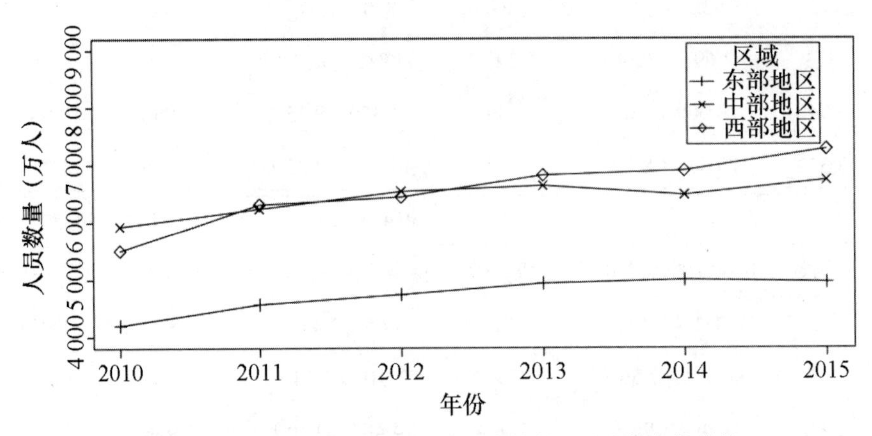

图 1　2010～2015 年不同地区传染病控制人员人数变化趋势

表 2　2010～2015 年不同地区传染病控制人员数量及其所占比例 [*n*（%）]

地区	2010 年	2011 年	2012 年	2013 年	2014 年	2015 年
东部	4 201（7.93）	4 567（8.10）	4 736（8.25）	4 925（8.30）	4 987（8.37）	4 946（8.44）
中部	5 929（8.16）	6 237（8.17）	6 537（8.28）	6 635（8.30）	6 474（8.27）	6 730（8.45）
西部	5 502（9.76）	6 308（9.93）	6 440（9.85）	6 816（9.91）	6 896（9.95）	7 269（9.82）

2.4 全国范围传染病控制人员与其他专业领域人员人数对比

2010～2015 年，每年传染病控制人员人数和比例均高于结核病控制和性病艾滋病防控的人员，其数量约是其他两个专业领域人数的 1.7～2.4 倍。但随着性病艾滋病防控人员人数的逐年递增，其数量与从事传染病控制的人员数量的差距正在逐渐缩小；但是结核病控制人员数量与传染病控制人员数量差距则逐年递增，见表 3。从不同级别疾控中心 3 种领域人员人数构成比来看，传染病控制人数构成比例，在每年的不同地区、不同级别的疾控中心中，均为最高。见表 4。

表 3　2010～2015 年全国疾控机构传染病控制、结核病防治以及性病艾滋病领域人员数量其所占比例 [*n*（%）]

专业	2010 年	2011 年	2012 年	2013 年	2014 年	2015 年
传染病控制	15 632（8.59）	17 112（8.72）	17 713（8.78）	18 376（8.83）	18 357（8.86）	18 945（8.92）
结核病防治	9 030（4.96）	9 537（4.86）	9 720（4.82）	9 688（4.66）	9 444（4.56）	9 342（4.40）
性病艾滋病	6 562（3.61）	8 386（4.27）	8 946（4.43）	9 380（4.51）	9 467（4.57）	9 966（4.69）

表 4　2010～2015 年各级疾控机构数及传染控制人员数、结核病防治人员数与艾滋病领域人员数及其所占比例 [*n*（%）]

级别	2010 年				2011 年			
	机构数	传染病控制人员数	结核病防治人员数	性病艾滋病领域人员数	机构数	传染病控制人员数	结核病防治人员数	性病艾滋病领域人员数
省级	32	932（7.62）	381（3.12）	536（4.38）	31	820（7.07）	307（2.65）	569（4.91）
地市级	353	2 691（7.29）	1 163（3.15）	1 389（3.76）	342	2 913（7.56）	1 192（3.09）	1 657（4.30）
区县级	2 948	12 009（9.04）	7 486（5.64）	4 637（3.49）	2 899	13 379（9.15）	8 038（5.50）	6 160（4.21）
合计	3 333	15 632（8.59）	9 030（4.96）	6 562（3.61）	3 272	17 112（8.72）	9 537（4.86）	8 386（4.27）

级别	2012 年				2013 年			
	机构数	传染病控制人员数	结核病防治人员数	性病艾滋病领域人员数	机构数	传染病控制人员数	结核病防治人员数	性病艾滋病领域人员数
省级	34	875（7.31）	321（2.68）	586（4.90）	32	861（7.24）	319（2.68）	577（4.85）
地市级	352	2 894（7.38）	1 168（2.98）	1 723（4.39）	347	3 021（7.56）	1 148（2.87）	1 758（4.39）
区县级	2 940	13 944（9.26）	8 231（5.47）	6 637（4.41）	2 972	14 494（9.28）	8 221（5.26）	7 047（4.51）
合计	3 326	17 713（8.78）	9 720（4.82）	8 946（4.43）	3 351	18 376（8.83）	9 688（4.66）	9 382（4.51）

续表

级别	2014年				2015年			
	机构数	传染病控制人员数	结核病防治人员数	性病艾滋病领域人员数	机构数	传染病控制人员数	结核病防治人员数	性病艾滋病领域人员数
省级	32	865（7.49）	305（2.64）	542（4.69）	32	888（7.38）	352（2.93）	567（4.71）
地市级	347	3 010（7.54）	1 125（2.82）	1 768(4.43）	348	3 045（7.61）	1 118（2.79）	1 801(4.50）
区县级	2 974	14 482(9.30）	8 014（5.15）	7 157(4.60）	2 966	15 012(9.37）	7 872（4.91）	7 598(4.74）
合计	3 353	18 357(8.86）	9 444（4.56）	9 467(4.57）	3 346	18 945(8.92）	9 342（4.40）	9 966(4.69）

2.5 新疆维吾尔自治区人员情况

总体来看，新疆维吾尔自治区疾控机构的人员中，受过大学本科及以上高等教育的人员比例自2011年起逐年增加（表5）。新疆省级疾控机构的传染病控制人员比例在2010～2012年有所增加，地市级疾控中心人员比例在2010～2015年间呈上下波动，区县级疾控中心人员比例较为稳定（图2）。结核病防控和性病艾滋病控制人员在各级疾控机构中的构成比在6年间均变化不大；2015年与2010年相比，新疆地区各级疾控机构的传染病控制人员比例均略有增加（表6）。与全国不同地区相比，新疆地区的省级疾控中心传染病防控人员所占比例在2012～2015年间，均低于东、中部地区，但高于西部地区；2010～2015年，其地市级疾控中心的比例均高于东、中部地区，但低于西部地区水平；区县级疾控中心的比例在6年间均高于东、中、西部地区；6年间，新疆的各级疾控中心的结核病防控与性病艾滋病控制人员比例均高于东、中、西部地区，见图2。

表5　2010～2015年新疆维吾尔自治区疾控机构人员学历构成（%）

学历	2010年	2011年	2012年	2013年	2014年	2015年
研究生	2.78	1.86	2.05	2.28	2.45	2.79
大学本科	35.91	23.87	24.23	25.20	26.59	27.42

表6　2010～2015年新疆传染病控制人员数量及其所占比例

项目	2010年		2011年		2012年		2013年		2014年		2015年	
	全国	新疆	全国	新疆	全国	新疆	全国	新疆	全国	新疆	全国	新疆
省级												
传染病控制人员人数	932（7.62）	36（6.91）	820（7.07）	36（6.91）	875（7.31）	37（7.54）	861（7.24）	34（7.56）	865（7.49）	34（7.49）	888（7.38）	34（7.49）

续表

项目	2010年		2011年		2012年		2013年		2014年		2015年	
	全国	新疆	全国	新疆	全国	新疆	全国	新疆	全国	新疆	全国	新疆
省级												
机构总人数	12 227	521	11 594	521	11 964	491	11 900	450	11 554	454	12 032	454
地市级												
传染病控制人员人数	2 691（7.29）	100（7.46）	2 913（7.56）	107（8.06）	2 894（7.38）	101（7.87）	3 021（7.56）	100（7.67）	3 010（7.54）	108（8.06）	3 045（7.61）	105（8.17）
机构总人数	36 924	1 340	38 548	1 328	39 216	1 284	39 966	1 304	39 923	1 340	40 004	1 285
区县级												
传染病控制人员人数	12 009（9.04）	359（11.08）	13 379（9.15）	386（11.40）	13 944（9.26）	402（11.74）	14 494（9.28）	405（11.56）	14 482（9.30）	411（11.47）	15 012（9.37）	412（11.59）
机构总人数	132 801	3 239	146 183	3 386	150 595	3 424	156 229	3 503	155 701	3 582	160 268	3 556
合计												
传染病控制人员人数	15 632（8.59）	495（9.71）	17 112（8.72）	529（10.11）	17 713（8.78）	540（10.39）	18 376（8.83）	539（10.25）	18 357（8.86）	553（10.29）	18 945（8.92）	551（10.41）
机构总人数	181 952	5 100	196 325	5 235	201 775	5 199	208 095	5 257	207 178	5 376	212 304	5 295

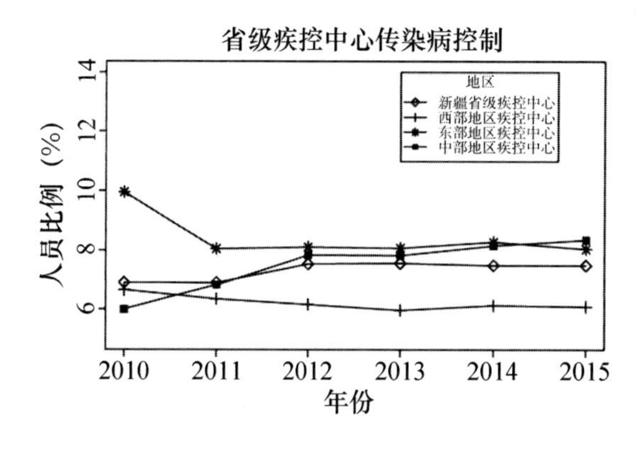

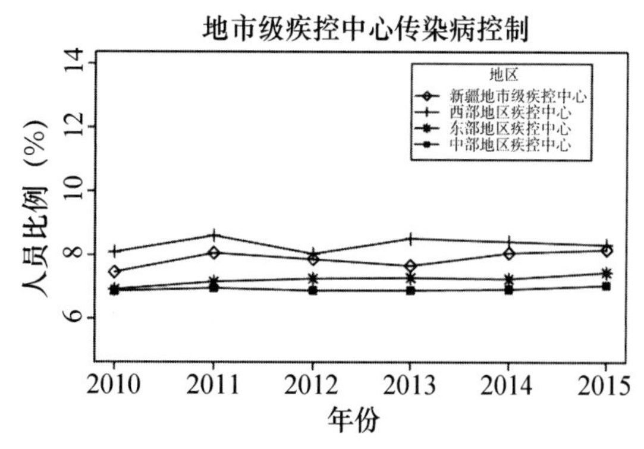

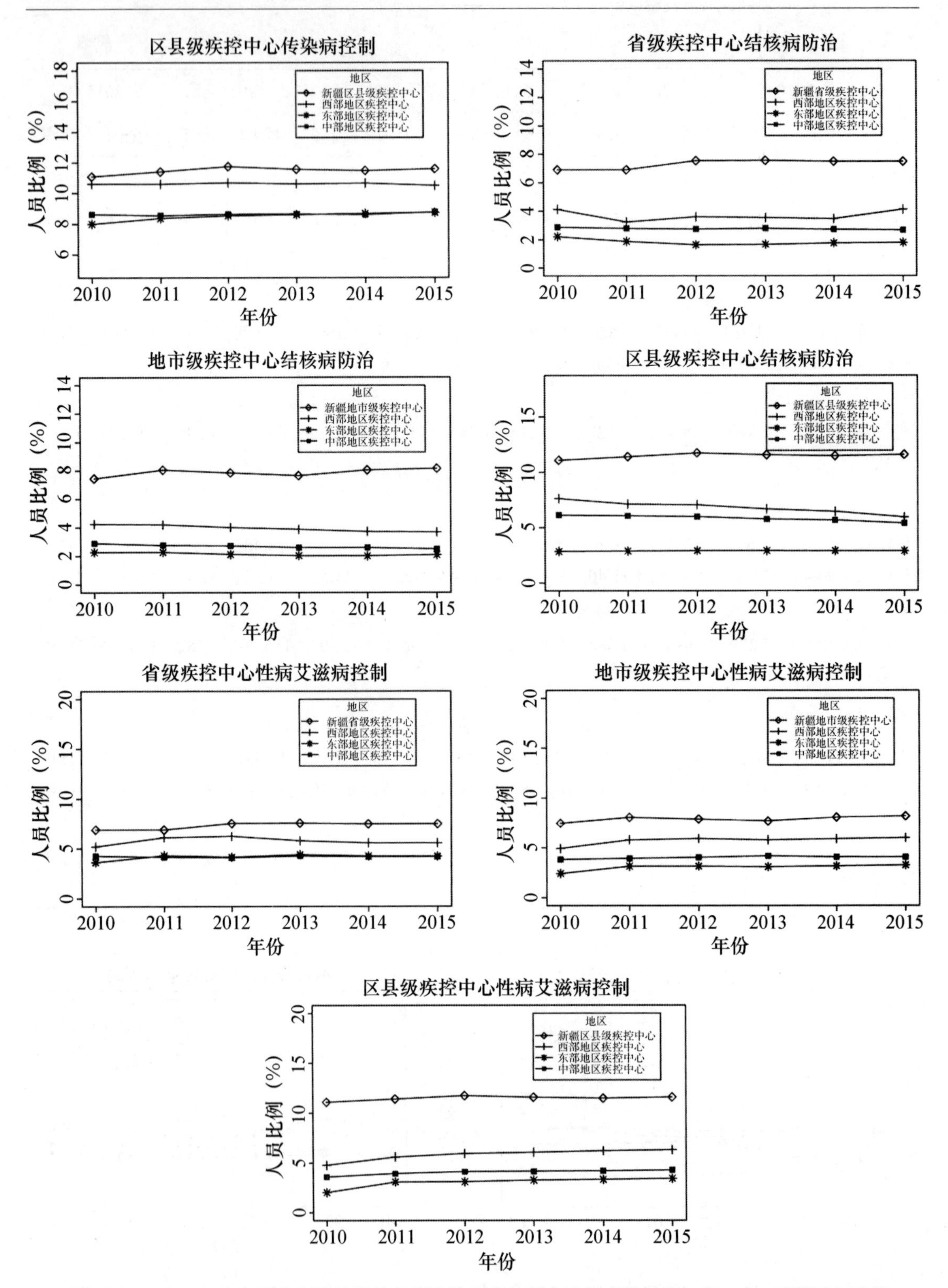

图 2　2010～2015 年新疆各级疾控机构传染病控制人员所占比例变化趋势与东、中、西部地区比较

2.6 全国不同地区传染病控制、结核病防治和性病艾滋病控制人员所占比例比较

图2还显示，在传染病控制领域，总体看来，除外2010～2011年东部地区省级疾控机构的大幅减少，以及2010～2012年间中部地区的大幅增加，6年间各地区人员比例趋势较为平稳。西部地区的地市级和区县级疾控中心人员比例历年均高于其他两个地区，但其省级疾控中心人员比例自2011年起总体呈现减少的趋势，并且低于其他两个地区。

在结核病防治领域，总体看来呈现西部地区人员比例最高，中部地区次之，东部地区比例最低的现象。西部地区的省级疾控机构人员比例在2015年有所增加，但该地区区县级疾控机构人员比例则在2015年略有减少；其余地区和级别的疾控机构人员比例在6年间变化不大。

在性病艾滋病控制领域，省级疾控机构中，2011～2015年东、中部地区从业人员比例极为接近，且6年间均低于西部地区的人员比例；地市级和区县级疾控中心与结核病防治人员比例在不同地区的分布情况相似，也呈现西部最高、中部次之、东部最低的情况。

3. 讨论

从总体情况来看，近年来，全国的传染病控制人员的人数以及全国所有疾控机构的人员总人数在逐年增加，新疆维吾尔自治区疾控机构和传染病控制人员人数和人员整体素质在提高。本研究在对比不同地区、不同级别疾控中心中三种专业领域人员人数构成比时发现，从全国总体情况来看，传染病控制人员与结核病防控和性病艾滋病领域防控从业人员相比，无论从数量上，还是从构成比例上看，均占有绝对的优势。新疆地区的传染病控制人员所占比例在6年间总体呈现增加的趋势，但是各级传染病控制人员比例与东、中、西部地区相比，并不占优势，尤其是区县级疾控中心。

研究还发现，尽管西部地区传染病控制人员人数比例高于东部和中部地区，但人员配比是否足够应付传染病控制的工作还需要其他的指标来辅助衡量。国家卫生计生委制定了《关于疾病预防控制机构岗位设置编制说明》[3]，并用“传染病控制岗位工作量权重系数”来评价疾控机构人员岗位编制的配比是否能够应对日程工作需要。本研究选取新疆维吾尔自治区作为研究对象，并对其传染病控制人员的情况进行了单独的分析。根据《关于疾病预防控制机构岗位设置编制说明》[3]中“传染病控制岗位工作量权重系数”的要求，传染病控制领域，省级、地市级和区县级疾控中心的权重系数分别为6.7、9.0和12.0。此权重系数分别对省、地市以及区县级别的不同专业领域岗位设置进行了要求。根据此权重系数的计算方法，数值越高说明工作量越大，则需要的人员数量也相应增加。2014年，新疆维吾尔自治区传染病控制人员的构成比分别为7.49%、8.06%、11.47%，比较相应的权重系数来看，新疆地市级和区县级疾控中心的传染病控制人员人数还需要再增加，而省级的人员数量也

应根据实际情况作出相应缩减。

尽管总体看来，中西部地区省级、地市级和区县级传染病控制领域人员近年来总体呈持续增长的趋势，这有利于增强当地传染病应对能力，特别是对于仍具有传染病暴发风险的新疆地区[4]，还应当补充当地疾控中心的防控人员。此外，从宏观的疾病控制角度考虑，由于新疆地区慢性心肺疾病现况和发展趋势日趋严重[5]，该地区正在同时面临传染病和慢性非传染性疾病的双重疾病负担，因此，为了更好的实现医防结合有效控制，在加强传染病防控人员配备的同时，也要考虑同时在疾控机构配备更多的慢性病防控相关专业人员。

致谢

感谢中国疾病预防控制中心对我工作上的支持，以及新疆维吾尔自治区疾病预防控制中心对本研究给予的帮助。特别感谢吴静老师为本文的写作方向提出宝贵的指导意见，提供相关的人力资源数据。同时感谢夏代提古丽·苏拉衣曼老师为本研究的写作提供的帮助和支持。

参考文献

[1] 武建国，司建林，孙富荣，等．2011～2012 年新疆和田地区法定管理新发传染病疫情分析 [J]．疾病预防控制通报，2013, 6: 29-31.

[2] 杨琼，司建林，王慧，等．2004～2011 年新疆和田地区法定传染病流行病学分析 [J]．疾病预防控制通报，2013, 3: 7-9, 16.

[3] 卫生部．关于疾病预防控制机构岗位设置编制说明 [R]．2012.

[4] 武建国，何晓兰，杨琼，等．2006～2011 年和田地区突发公共卫生事件及法定传染病疫情信息分析 [J]．疾病预防控制通报，2012, 5: 62-64, 84.

[5] 陈海英，刘继文，张静．新疆慢性非传染性疾病相关危险因素的调查研究 [J]．医药前沿，2012, 20: 39-40.

我国疾病预防控制机构实验室检验能力分析△

米玉倩，吴　静，梁晓峰

中国疾病预防控制中心，北京 102206

通讯作者：梁晓峰。E-mail：liangxf@ hotmail.com

摘　要　目的　了解我国各级疾控机构在实验室检验能力方面的建设情况，找出存在的问题并提出建议。**方法**　采用描述性流行病学研究方法，利用 SAS 9.2 软件和 Excel 2010 进行统计学分析和趋势分析。**结果**　我国各级疾控中心卫生检验人数及比例总体呈上升趋势；专用实验室数量在 2012 年增幅较大，之后增长速度放缓；实验室仪器设备拥有率在 2011 年急剧增加后趋于平稳，东部地区各级疾控中心平均拥有实验室仪器设备数量均高于中、西部地区；省、县区级疾控中心基本检验项目达标率东部最高、中部次之、西部最低，而地市级疾控中心基本检验项目达标率中部最高、东部次之、西部最低。**结论**　我国各级疾控机构卫生检验人员素质还有待进一步提升。省级疾控中心实验室仪器设备拥有率与地市、县区级相比在数量上处于绝对优势。我国东、中部疾控中心检验项目开展相对较好，而西部地区比较薄弱。省级疾控机构实验室检验和诊断项目在数量方面地区均衡性和公平性最好。

关键词　疾病预防控制；实验室；检验能力

Analysis on the Chinese disease control and prevention institutions' laboratory testing capacity

Mi Yuqian, Wu Jing, Liang Xiaofeng

Chinese Center for Disease Control and Prevention, Beijing 102206, China

Abstract　Objective　The objective of this study is to understand the construction of laboratory testing capacity of the Chinese Disease Control and Prevention institutions at all levels and to expound the problems and puts

△　本文发表于：中国卫生政策研究，2017，10（3）：75-80.

forward the related suggestions and countermeasures which can provide the basis for scientific and corresponding improvement of laboratory construction. **Methods** The whole procedures were completed through descriptive epidemiological studies using SAS 9.2 Software and Excel 2010 for conducting statistical and trend analyses. **Results** There was an increasing trend in the number and proportion of inspections in the disease control institutions at all levels in China. The number of disease control and prevention institutions' special testing laboratories increased significantly in 2012 and then the growth rate slowed down. The owning rate of equipped laboratory appliance rapidly rose in 2011 and then began to level off. The average number of equipment in eastern region was greater than that drawn in the central and western regions. According to rate of compliance with the standard of basic laboratory projects, there was a trend in the provincial, district, and county level disease control and prevention institutions where the eastern region came first, followed by the central region and the western region. However, in general, this rate of those provincial level institutions showed a state that the central region holds the highest rate, the eastern region comes second, and the western last. **Conclusions** The qualities of health inspection personnel still need to be further improved in disease control and prevention institutions at all levels in the country. In the aspect of laboratory equipment possession rate, the provincial CDCs have greater and absolute advantage than the county-level and district level institutions. The testing projects of CDCs in the central and eastern regions of China have a relatively good level, while those tracked in the western region are relatively weak. China should strengthen the support to western region in terms of human resource, equipment and funding. The provincial-level disease control and prevention institutions' laboratory testing and diagnosis projects are the best in balance and fairness. Improving the testing capacity is an effective approach to promote the development of disease control and prevention. Hence, the state should pay much attention to the laboratory construction works and management strategies and flows.

Key words Disease control and prevention; laboratory; testing capacity

实验室检验能力是一个综合性指标，与人员、设备、经费等因素有着密切的联系。实验室仪器设备装备和检验检测水平是疾病预防控制体系建设的重要组成部分。实验室检测、分析与评价作为疾控机构的核心职能之一，承担着卫生防疫、卫生监督监测、健康相关产品卫生质量检测和评价、食品安全风险监测及评估的重要职责，尤其为疾病防控、突发公共卫生事件应急处置提供了重要的技术支撑[1]。近年来新发传染病增多、旧式传染病死灰复燃，疾控机构实验室检测的准确度与时效性作为整个实验室检验能力的基础，直接关系到疫情和事件的处置效果。本研究通过对 2010 ~ 2014 年我国各级疾控机构卫生检验人员状况、专用实验室配备情况、实验室检验仪器拥有情况、基本检验项目开展情况进行描述性统计，对全国各级疾控机构实验室检验能力建设情况作出分析、评估，以期为卫生行政部门掌控疾控资源、制定能力提升方案和行动规划提供数据支持。

1. 资料与方法

1.1 资料来源

通过我国疾病预防控制基本信息年度报告系统收集 2010 ~ 2014 年全国省级、地市级、县区级疾控中心卫生检验人员状况、专用实验室配备情况、实验室仪器设备拥有情况和基本检验项目开展情况。

1.2 研究方法

用 Excel 2010 软件建立数据库，采用 SAS9.2 软件和 Excel 2010 对数据进行分析。对原始数据进行再次逻辑核对后，分不同时间、不同地区、不同层级，对疾控机构卫生检验人员状况、专用实验室数量、设备装备和检验项目开展情况等进行描述性统计分析和趋势分析。

2. 结果

2.1 卫生检验人员状况

从全国疾病预防控制机构人员具有的执业资质范围分布情况看，以公共卫生和检验技术人员为主，截至 2015 年 7 月 1 日，共有 71 506 人，其中卫生检验技术人员占 12.43%。全国疾病预防控制机构人员主要执业范围分布在环境卫生等五大卫生、传染病控制、计划免疫和卫生检验这四个范围，其中卫生检验的人员比例为 7.93%。2011 ~ 2014 年我国各级疾控中心卫生检验人数及比例均呈上升趋势，省级卫生检验人数及比例在 2014 年略有下降（表 1）。

表 1　2011 ~ 2014 年全国各级疾控中心卫生检验人员情况

年份	省级疾控中心		地市级疾控中心		县区级疾控中心	
	人数	比例（%）	人数	比例（%）	人数	比例（%）
2011	915	7.89	2 621	6.8	7 040	4.82
2012	1 050	8.78	3 296	8.4	8 805	5.85
2013	1 241	10.43	4 016	10.05	10 265	6.57
2014	1 165	10.08	4 239	10.62	11 019	7.08

2.2 专用实验室配备情况

2014 年全国共报告专用实验室 10 170 个。总体来看，我国各级疾控中心专用实验室数量在 2012 年增幅较大，之后增长速度放缓。地市级疾控中心专用实验室数量由西部最多、中部次之、东部最少转变为西部最多、东部次之、中部最少。县区级疾控中心中部地区拥有专用实验室数量最多，东部次之，西部最少。省级、地市级疾控中心 P2 实验室（即二级生物安全防护实验室）数量最多，县区级疾控中心拥有艾滋病初筛实验室数量最多。P3 实验室（即三级生物安全防护实验室）主要分布在东部省级疾控中心和西部县区级疾控中心（表 2）。

表 2　2011～2014 年全国东中西部疾病预防控制中心专用实验室拥有情况

年份	地区	P3 实验室	1 000 级净化实验室	局部 100 级	P2 实验室	脊灰确认实验室	艾滋病确认实验室	艾滋病初筛实验室	微生物检验	理化检验	毒理实验	其他
2011	省级	12	36	12	140	24	24	11	7	9	6	13
	东部地区	7	9	2	38	9	9	6	1	1	1	~
	中部地区	4	16	4	51	8	7	2	3	4	3	4
	西部地区	1	11	6	51	7	8	3	3	4	2	9
	地市级	3	234	81	486	7	191	208	37	38	4	33
	东部地区	3	80	20	143	4	51	48	9	8	3	7
	中部地区	—	107	28	187	3	74	77	18	20	1	14
	西部地区	—	47	33	156	—	66	83	10	10	—	12
	县区级	36	480	172	1 001	22	62	2 328	227	251	24	147
	东部地区	11	197	51	327	12	17	593	47	70	1	32
	中部地区	9	199	59	367	3	25	879	98	100	14	52
	西部地区	16	84	62	307	7	20	856	82	81	9	63
2012	省级	14	23	13	134	26	22	15	64	70	27	56
	东部地区	7	8	2	59	8	9	5	11	23	14	14
	中部地区	4	7	7	37	11	7	3	11	11	8	27
	西部地区	3	8	4	38	7	6	7	42	36	5	15
	地市级	6	184	142	485	3	230	186	202	186	12	139

续表

年份	地区	P3 实验室	1 000 级净化实验室	局部 100 级	P2 实验室	脊灰确认实验室	艾滋病确认实验室	艾滋病初筛实验室	微生物检验	理化检验	毒理实验	其他
	东部地区	2	63	44	132	2	59	43	34	35	5	26
	中部地区	2	80	60	186	1	88	73	93	80	4	55
	西部地区	2	41	38	167	—	83	70	75	71	3	58
	县区级	29	368	234	1 055	—	98	2 274	1 027	1 048	90	565
	东部地区	6	77	43	310	—	17	606	260	282	27	94
	中部地区	5	240	139	446	—	44	910	405	409	38	199
	西部地区	18	51	52	299	—	37	758	362	357	25	272
2013	省级	14	27	17	178	28	24	15	76	89	52	112
	东部地区	8	9	4	95	9	9	4	12	25	16	31
	中部地区	3	10	7	42	10	7	3	22	31	31	63
	西部地区	3	8	6	41	9	8	8	42	33	5	18
	地市级	4	174	155	514	3	239	179	241	271	14	160
	东部地区	2	59	58	165	1	76	46	49	50	6	44
	中部地区	1	77	55	172	2	80	63	105	136	4	54
	西部地区	1	38	42	177	—	83	70	87	85	4	62
	县区级	21	360	265	1 096	—	100	2 322	1 200	1 222	89	660
	东部地区	1	145	109	464	—	26	759	363	365	21	157
	中部地区	5	160	98	307	—	39	719	413	440	41	168
	西部地区	15	55	58	325	—	35	844	424	417	27	335
2014	省级	14	26	16	176	26	24	13	79	92	53	118
	东部地区	8	9	4	95	9	9	4	13	25	16	31
	中部地区	4	10	7	43	9	6	3	22	31	31	64
	西部地区	2	7	5	38	8	9	6	44	36	6	23
	地市级	4	173	157	514	3	238	173	239	283	15	166
	东部地区	1	60	61	166	1	77	43	56	61	7	41

续表

年份	地区	P3 实验室	1 000 级净化实验室	局部 100 级	P2 实验室	脊灰确认实验室	艾滋病确认实验室	艾滋病初筛实验室	微生物检验	理化检验	毒理实验	其他
	中部地区	2	76	52	169	2	78	61	104	138	4	58
	西部地区	1	37	44	179	—	83	69	79	84	4	67
	县区级	21	352	283	1 092	—	107	2 269	1 300	1 336	84	724
	东部地区	2	141	120	474	—	26	752	412	434	20	172
	中部地区	5	157	105	298	—	39	697	429	453	39	186
	西部地区	14	54	58	320	—	42	820	459	449	25	366

2.3 实验室仪器设备拥有情况

2010～2014 年，我国东部地区各级疾控中心平均拥有实验室仪器设备数量均高于中部地区和西部地区。省级疾控中心平均拥有实验室仪器设备数量除 2011 年外，西部地区均高于中部地区。地市级疾控中心平均拥有实验室仪器设备数量中部地区高于西部地区。县区级疾控中心平均拥有实验室仪器设备数量除 2012 年中部地区略低于西部地区外，其余年份中部地区高于西部地区（图 1）。

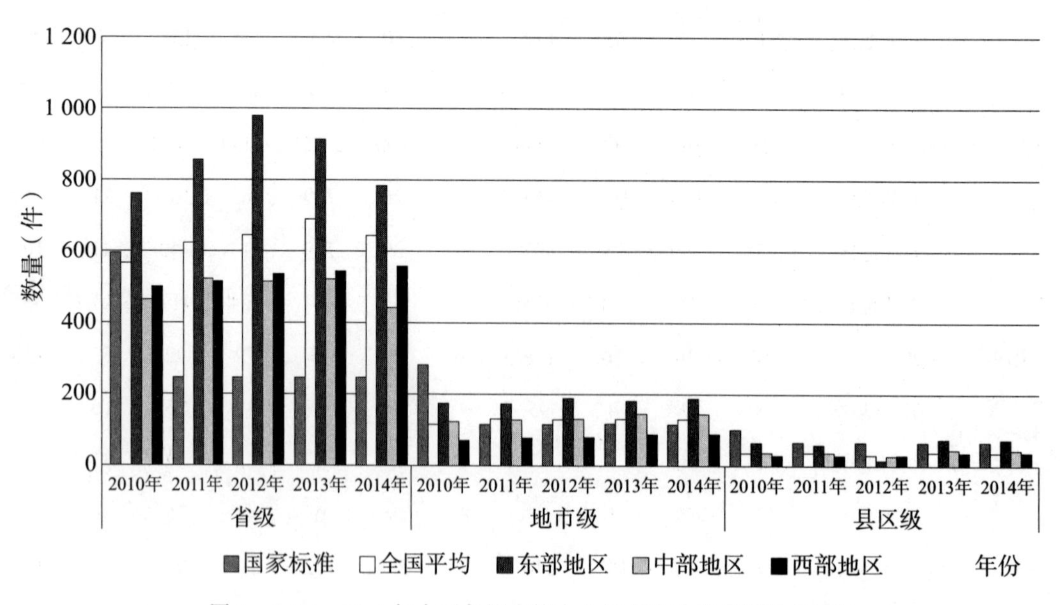

图 1　2010～2014 年全国各级疾控中心拥有实验室仪器设备情况

五年间全国各级疾控中心实验室仪器设备拥有率大致呈现2011年急剧增加，之后趋于平稳的态势。这是由于2011年我国采用了新的仪器设备配置标准，所以各级疾控中心实验室设备拥有率较2010年相比均有大幅的提高（图2）。

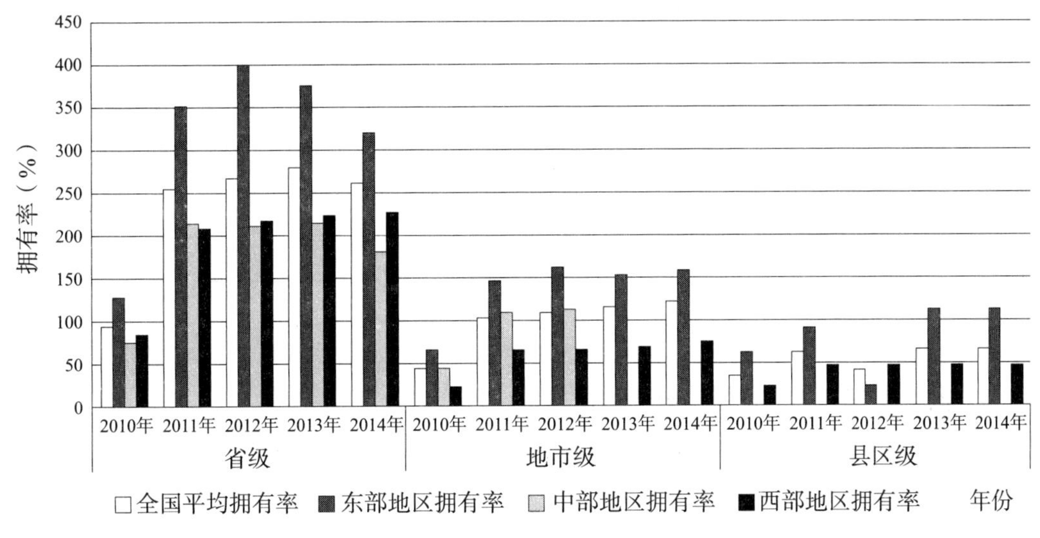

图2 2010～2014年全国各级疾控中心平均实验室仪器设备拥有率

2.4 基本检验项目开展情况

总体来看，疾控中心基本检验项目达标率省级最高，地市级次之，县区级最低。五年间，省级、地市级、县区级疾控中心与国家标准的平均差额分别为105项、79项、55项。由于2011年各级疾控中心上调检验项目的国家标准，省级、地市级、县区级疾控中心基本检验项的国家标准分别由2010年的379项调整为387项、224项调整为226项、116项调整为118项，故2011年各级疾控中心基本检验项目达标率出现下降。2011～2014年省级疾控中心平均检验项增减幅度不大，2014年出现上升趋势；2011～2013年地市级疾控中心平均检验项逐渐增高，2014年比2013年略有降低；县区级疾控中心基本检验项目达标率在2012～2014年间基本持平（图3）。

观察五年间全国东、中、西部疾控中心基本检验项目达标情况可知（图4），省、县区级疾控中心基本检验项目达标率呈现东部最高、中部次之、西部最低的总体特征，而地市级疾控中心基本检验项目达标率中部最高、东部次之、西部最低。中部各级疾控中心达标率标准差最小，地市级疾控中心与省级疾控中心基本检验项目达标率相近，县区级疾控中心基本检验项目达标率略低。东部地区省、地市、县区三级疾控中心基本检验项平均差额2011年最多，为84项，2010年最少，为45项；中部地区省、地市、县区三级疾控中心基本检验项平均差额2012年最多，为75项，2011年最少，为69项；西部地区省、地市、县区三级疾控中心基本检验项平均差额 2014 年最多，为 118 项，2010 年最少，为 91 项。

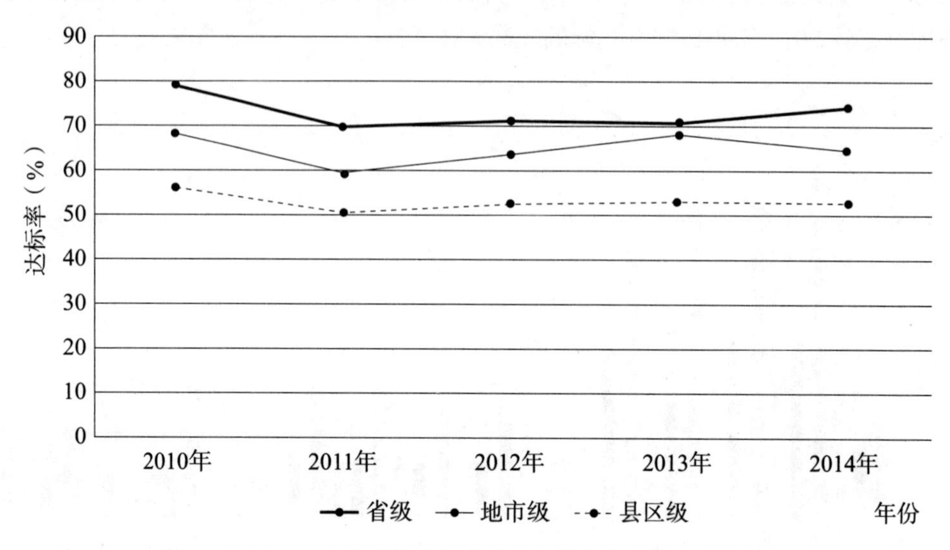

图 3　2010～2014 年全国各级疾控中心基本检验项目达标情况

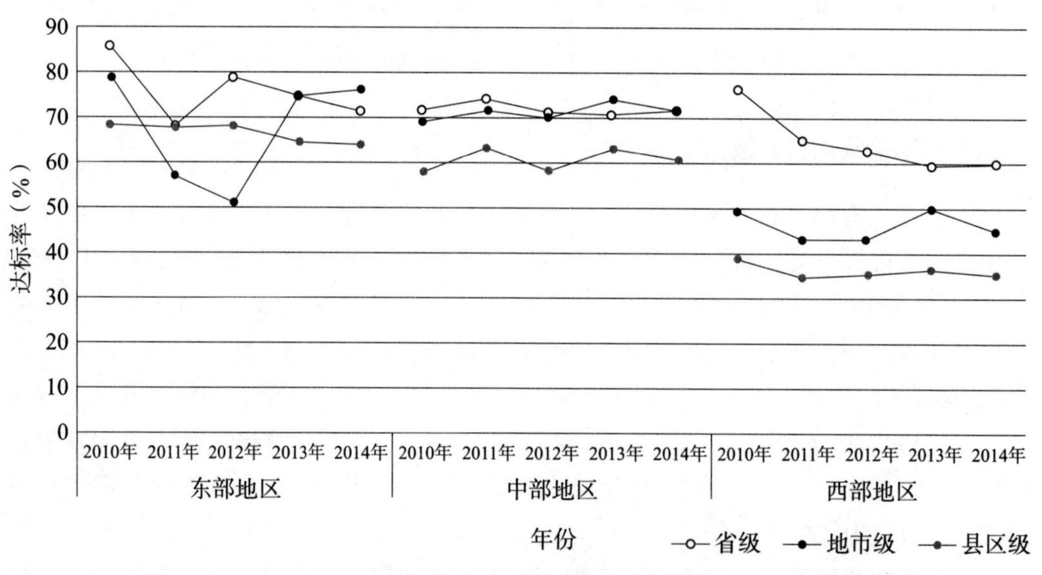

图 4　2010～2014 年全国东、中、西部疾控中心检验能力达标情况

3. 讨论

近年来，实验室检验检测在控制新旧传染病的暴发流行中发挥了至关重要的作用，世界范围内频繁发生的重大突发公共卫生事件也对实验室检验能力提出了更高的要求[2]。

H5N1 型禽流感病毒自 2004 年开始肆虐亚洲各国，2010 年发端于北美洲的甲型 H1N1 流感疫情在全球蔓延，埃博拉疫情于 2013 年在几内亚暴发。对这些传染病开展有效的防控工作，都离不开疾控机构实验室的技术支持。随着食品安全、饮用水安全、环境污染等问题引起越来越多的关注，加强疾控机构实验室建设也成为我国公共卫生体系应急能力的重点，实验室装备和检验能力建设已成为疾病预防控制体系的重要组成部分，也成为衡量疾病预防控制机构技术水平、工作能力的重要标志[3]。2003 年 SARS 疫情暴发以来，国家和各级地方政府对疾控机构的实验室建设加大了投入。2004 年全国各级疾控中心按照国家卫生计生委、国家发展改革委《省、地、县级疾病预防控制中心实验室建设指导意见》的要求，进一步加强了实验室设备投入和仪器配置[4]，改善了实验室基础设施和环境条件，增添了部分先进的检测设备，加强了实验室质量管理，检验能力得到大大提高。

卫生检验人员作为推动疾病预防控制中心持续发展的技术人才，对实验室检验功能与检验成果有着直接的影响[5]。2011 ~ 2014 年全国各级疾控中心卫生检验人员数量及比例逐年增长，标志着疾控队伍逐渐壮大与持续发展。但疾控机构人员学历层次偏低，提示政府应当加大投入，提高福利性待遇水平、创造良好的工作环境与学习、培训、进修条件来吸引高学历、高素质的卫生检验人才。

实验室仪器设备配置水平直观上反映了疾病预防控制体系的建设成效，今后仍需将实验室仪器设备作为机构运行的硬件基础予以重视，既要确保疾病预防控制、突发公共卫生事件应急处置、公共卫生监督等检验检测工作的顺利开展，又要避免仪器设备的重复购置、资源浪费、配置不均。五年间省级疾控中心拥有的实验室仪器设备远超地市和县区级疾控中心，在数量上处于绝对优势。省级实验室仪器设备配置较高对于省级疾控机构承担地市级、县区级疾控中心实验室检验检测与评价职能具有重要作用。拥有专用实验室的地市级疾控中心数量在逐年上升，部分地市级疾控中心的实验室拥有情况已经接近省级配置。《省、地、县级疾病预防控制中心实验室建设指导意见》中也明确提出了实验室建设要有力地推动硬件建设和实验室规范化建设与发展。

2014 年省级疾控中心平均检验项目数量出现上升，省级疾控中心检验项目达标率最高的是四川省，达到了 94.57%；2011 ~ 2013 年地市级疾控中心平均检验项大体逐年升高，由此反映了国家对加强基础检验能力建设的重视。我国东部、中部地区疾控中心检验项目开展相对较好，省、地市、县区三级疾控中心平均检验项均高于全国平均水平，而西部地区比较薄弱，低于全国平均水平，西部县区级疾控中心在 2014 年检验项目达标率仅为 35.79%。由此可见，国家仍旧需要加大对西部地区疾控中心的扶持力度。省级疾控机构实验室检验和诊断项目数量方面，其地区均衡性和公平性最好。从相对均衡性上来看，省级优于地市级、地市级优于县区级，提示受地方财政的影响，政府对地市、县区两级机构的投入明显低于省级的投入水平，应该在今后予以充分地关注。总体来看，各级疾控中心平均检验项目数都达不到国家标准的八成，其可能原因是某些疾病不存在或者已被很好的控制因此没有开展某些检验项目的需要，抑或该检验项目的开展需要很高的维持成本而未开展[5]，这也提示政策制定者应考虑当地实际需要和能力、分地域、按经济发展水平制定更为适合的检验项目开展标准。

参考文献

[1] 王勤．淄博市疾病控制机构卫生检验资源配置现状与检验能力评价研究 [D]．济南：山东大学，2010.

[2] 王锡辉．广州市区县疾病预防控制机构实验室检验能力现状及评价 [D]．广州：中山大学，2009.

[3] 王海红．东营市疾病预防控制机构实验室能力建设现状分析 [D]．济南 : 山东大学，2015.

[4] 柴煜卿．我国疾病预防控制机构实验室检验能力评价研究 [D]．上海：复旦大学，2008.

[5] 顾燕玲．疾病预防控制中心卫生检验能力现状与发展 [J]．中国校医，2015(11)：863-864.

2011～2015年我国疾病预防控制机构仪器设备配置状况△

王嘉艺[1]，吴　静[2]，王学梅[1]

1. 内蒙古医科大学公共卫生学院，呼和浩特 010110；2. 中国疾病预防控制中心慢病社区处
通信作者：吴静，Email：wujingcdc@163.com

摘　要　目的　了解2011～2015年我国不同层级、不同地区疾控机构仪器设备配置变化情况，为制订疾控体系仪器设备配置规划提供依据。**方法**　通过全国疾控基本信息统计分析报告收集原始数据，运用Excel 2010整理分析数据，对全国疾控机构仪器设备的配置情况分层级、年度、地区、设备种类进行统计学描述和变化趋势分析。**结果**　2011～2015年全国各层级、各地区的疾控机构仪器设备平均拥有数量与达标率总体呈逐年增加的趋势。省级疾控机构仪器设备的配置总数远远超过国家标准，而地市级西部地区与县区级中、西部地区的疾控机构均未达标，全国疾控机构仪器设备配置表现出不均衡性。从仪器设备的分类项目看，不同级别和地区疾控机构有不同种类的配置缺乏情况，地市、县区级疾控机构普遍对健康教育器材的配置较低，地市、县区级的西部地区疾控机构对所有项目的仪器设备配置均未达标。**结论**　我国基层和西部地区疾控机构仪器设备的配置仍需增加，并应增强对健康教育器材配置的重视，从要求与需求的实际出发，合理完善疾控体系仪器设备的配置建设。

关键词　疾控机构；仪器设备；配置；达标率

The Allocation of Instrument and Equipment in Disease Control and Prevention Institutions in China (2011-2015)

Wang Jiayi[1], Wu Jing[2], Wang Xuemei[1]

1. Inner Mongolia Medical University, Hohhot, Inner Mongolia 010110, China

2. Chinese Center for Disease Control and Prevention, Beijing 102206, china

Corresponding author: WU Jing, Email: wujingcdc@163. com

△　本文发表于：公共卫生与预防医学，2017，28（3）：22-26.

Abstract **Objective** To understand the allocation of the instrument and equipment at different levels and in different regions of China from 2011-2015, and provide evidence for the allocation plan of instrument and equipment for the CDC system. **Methods** The original data about the instrument and equipment allocation were collected from the national CDC statistical analysis report. Excel 2010 was used to manage and analyze the data, statistical description and trend analysis was performed for the allocation of instrument and equipment at different levels, in different regions and years, types were also classified. **Results** There was an increasing trend of the average number and standard reaching the rate of instrument and equipment at all levels and in all regions of CDC from 2011 to 2015 in China. Additionally, at the provincial level of CDC, this number even exceeded the national standard. However, in the municipal CDCs in the central and western region and the county, the results did not reach the national standard. Overall, the allocation of the instrument and equipment were not balanced in the whole country. Furthermore, according to the classification of instruments and equipment, There were deficiencies of instruments and equipment at different levels and in different regions of CDCs. The standard reaching rate of health education instruments was low at grassroots level of CDCs. In the western region of CDCs, the allocation of all kinds of instrument and equipment did not reach the national standard. **Conclusions** The government should increase the allocation number of instrument and equipment to the grassroots and the western region of CDCs. Moreover, more attention should be paid to the allocation of health education instruments. In a word, the reasonable allocation of the equipment and instrument in China should be based on the practical requirement and demand.

Key words Disease control and prevention institutions; Instruments and equipment; Allocation; The standard reaching rate

疾病预防控制（疾控）机构承担着保障人民群众健康的重要职责，涵盖传染病、慢性病、健康教育等多方面任务，是政府实施公共卫生职能的专业机构[1，2]。而仪器设备作为疾控机构的硬件设施，是疾控机构完成工作任务和开展检测项目的基本条件，同时还影响着疾控机构科研与教育培训的水平，其配置与疾控工作能力密切相关，是疾控体系建设的重要内容之一[3，4]。随着国家对疾控机构的投入逐年增加，基础设施已日益改善[5]，但对仪器设备的配置投入是否合理、全国各级各地区的发展水平是否一致还需进行全面的了解。对2011～2015年期间我国疾控机构仪器设备配置情况进行分析，以了解不同层级、不同地区的疾控机构仪器设备配置五年变化趋势，为客观评估疾控体系当前的硬件基础建设进展和为今后制订疾控机构仪器设备配置规划提供科学依据。

1. 资料与方法

1.1 资料来源

来自2011～2015年全国疾病预防控制基本信息统计分析报告，收集其中全国省级、地市级、县区级疾控中心五年仪器设备配置信息。该报告系统覆盖全国各省、地市、县区级疾控机构，由接受过统一培训的工作人员在线填报信息，2011～2015 年每年仪器设备信息的报告率均达 90.00% 以上，5 年内报告率未达到 90.00% 的省份中几乎都有西藏、江西和内蒙古。信息上报后经过中国疾控中心严格审查与核对，研究收集的数据真实可靠。

1.2 分析方法

数据收集后再次进行逻辑核对，并用 Excel 2010 软件整理及分析数据。按层级、年度、地区、设备种类分类，对全国疾控机构的仪器设备配置数量信息进行统计学描述和趋势分析。

2. 结果

2.1 全国疾控机构仪器设备配置基本状况

五年间省级、地市级、县区级疾控机构平均拥有仪器设备数量都有一定的增加。省级疾控机构从 2011 年的仪器设备合计平均拥有件数 1 130 件，到 2015 年增加为 1 442 件；地市级疾控机构从 2011 年平均拥有 214 件，到 2015 年增加为 250 件；县区级疾控机构从 2011 年平均拥有 59 件，到 2015 年增加为 70 件。

省级、地市级、县区级疾控机构总仪器设备的达标率也逐年升高（图 1），但各级别的达标水平却有所不同。省级疾控机构五年间仪器设备平均拥有数量均远远超过国家标准；地市级疾控机构在 2013 年才实现达标；而县区级疾控机构达标率虽然逐年上升，但一直未达到国家标准，截至 2015 年达标率仍为 66.04%。

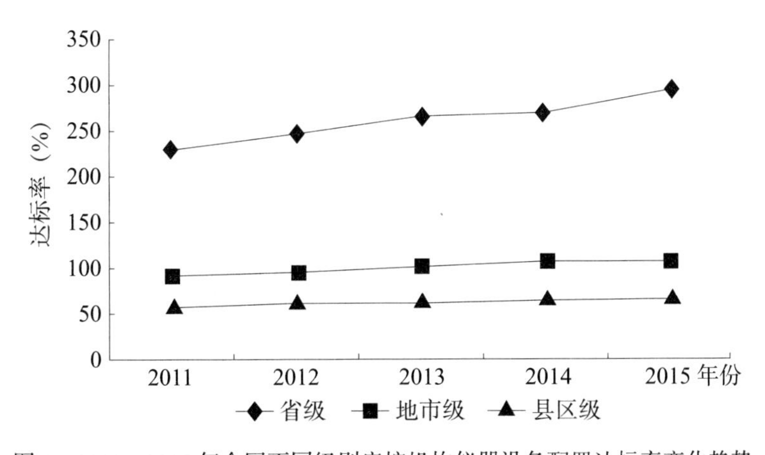

图 1 2011～2015 年全国不同级别疾控机构仪器设备配置达标率变化趋势

按照仪器设备的项目，可分为实验室仪器设备、健康教育器材、信息设备、车辆和冷链设备及器材。五年间省级疾控机构五种项目设备的配置都远远达标，截至 2015 年达标率最高者为信息设备，其平均拥有数量为国家标准的3.76倍；地市级疾控机构截至2015年对健康教育器材、车辆和冷链设备及器材的配置还未达标；县区级疾控机构截至2015年对实验室仪器设备、健康教育器材、信息设备的配置还未达标，尤其是对健康教育器材的配置较少，2015年达标率仅为25.00%（表1）。

表1　2011～2015年全国不同级别项目疾控机构仪器设备配置状况

仪器设备	国家标准	2011年		2012年		2013年		2014年		2015年	
		平均拥有件数	达标率（%）	平均拥有件数	达标率（%）	平均拥有件数	达标率（%）	平均拥有件数	达标率（%）	平均拥有件数	达标率（%）
省级											
实验室仪器设备	244	620	254.10	653	267.62	688	281.97	647	265.16	723	296.31
健康教育器材	54	57	105.56	63	116.67	69	127.78	71	131.48	74	137.04
信息设备	149	371	248.99	417	279.87	470	315.44	531	356.38	560	375.84
车辆	14	20	142.86	18	128.57	19	135.71	19	135.71	19	135.71
冷链设备及器材	31	62	200.00	52	167.74	56	180.65	61	196.77	66	212.90
地市级											
实验室仪器设备	115	121	105.22	128	111.30	135	117.39	139	120.87	138	120.00
健康教育器材	30	11	36.67	12	40.00	12	40.00	13	43.33	12	40.00
信息设备	67	62	92.54	68	101.49	74	110.45	80	119.40	80	119.40
车辆	7	6	85.71	5	71.43	6	85.71	6	85.71	5	71.43
冷链设备及器材	17	14	82.35	15	88.24	14	82.35	15	88.24	15	88.24
县区级											
实验室仪器设备	61	37	60.66	39	63.93	40	65.57	41	67.21	42	68.85
健康教育器材	12	3	25.00	3	25.00	3	25.00	3	25.00	3	25.00
信息设备	25	12	48.00	14	56.00	15	60.00	16	64.00	17	68.00
车辆	2	2	100.00	2	100.00	2	100.00	2	100.00	2	100.00
冷链设备及器材	6	5	83.33	6	100.00	6	100.00	6	100.00	6	100.00

2.2 省级不同地区疾控机构仪器设备配置状况

2015 年全国省级实报信息的疾控机构共有 31 个。据数据显示，2011～2015 年间东部、中部、西部地区的省级疾控机构仪器设备平均拥有数量均达到国家标准（表 2），其中东部地区最多，其次为西部，最后为中部。从仪器设备的分类项目来看，5 年间，东部、中部地区省级疾控机构所有项目仪器设备的配置均达到了国家标准，尤以信息设备和实验室仪器设备的达标率较高，远超国家标准 2～4 倍，而西部地区仅冷链设备及器材配置还未达标，截至 2015 年达标率为 96.77%，其余项目均达标。

表 2　2011～2015 年省级不同地区疾控机构仪器设备配置状况

地区	2011 年		2012 年		2013 年		2014 年		2015 年	
	平均拥有件数	达标率（%）	平均拥有件数	达标率（%）	平均拥有件数	达标率（%）	平均拥有件数	达标率（%）	平均拥有件数	达标率（%）
国家标准	492	100.00	492	100.00	492	100.00	492	100.00	492	100.00
东部	1 465	297.76	1 679	341.26	1 617	328.66	1 526	310.16	1 904	386.99
中部	975	198.17	959	194.92	977	198.58	882	179.27	907	184.35
西部	997	202.64	1 057	214.84	1 135	230.69	1 226	249.19	1 261	256.30

2.3 地市级不同地区疾控机构仪器设备配置状况

2015 年全国地市级实报信息的疾控机构数共 334 个。据 2011～2015 年每年上报的数据，可见地市级疾控机构仪器设备平均拥有数量逐年呈小幅增加趋势（表 3），东部、中部地区到 2015 年都达到了国家标准，唯有西部地区未达标。从仪器设备的分类项目来看，东部地区的疾控机构实验室仪器设备与信息设备的配置达标率较高，健康教育器材达标率较低；中部地区疾控机构截至 2015 年，健康教育器材与车辆的配置仍未达到国家标准（图 2）；而西部地区疾控机构五年间所有项目的仪器设备配置均未达到国家标准。

表 3　2011～2015 年地市级不同地区疾控机构仪器设备配置状况

地区	2011 年		2012 年		2013 年		2014 年		2015 年	
	平均拥有件数	达标率（%）	平均拥有件数	达标率（%）	平均拥有件数	达标率（%）	平均拥有件数	达标率（%）	平均拥有件数	达标率（%）
国家标准	236	100.00	236	100.00	236	100.00	236	100.00	236	100.00
东部	300	127.12	326	138.14	325	137.71	334	141.53	325	137.71

续表

地区	2011 年		2012 年		2013 年		2014 年		2015 年	
	平均拥有件数	达标率（%）	平均拥有件数	达标率（%）	平均拥有件数	达标率（%）	平均拥有件数	达标率（%）	平均拥有件数	达标率（%）
中部	225	95.34	239	101.27	255	108.05	269	113.98	269	113.98
西部	127	53.81	129	54.66	145	61.44	152	64.41	162	68.64

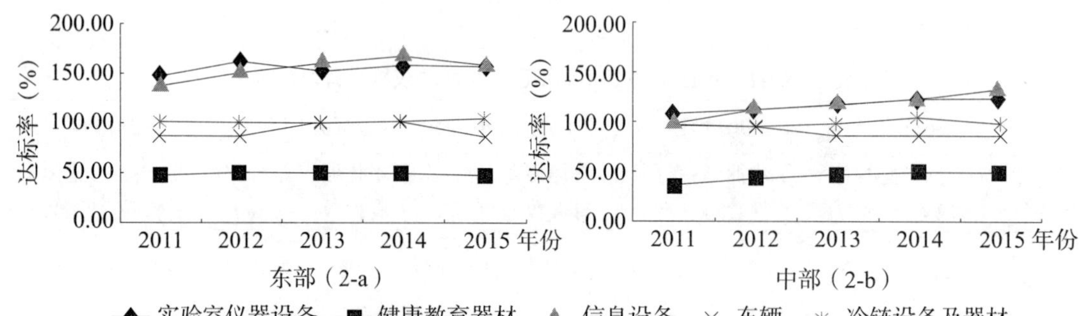

图 2　2011 ~ 2015 年地市级不同东、中部地区疾控机构五项仪器设备配置达标率变化趋势

2.4　县区级不同地区疾控机构仪器设备配置状况

2015 年全国县区级实报信息的疾控机构数共 2 777 个。县区级不同地区的疾控机构仪器设备平均拥有数量逐年增加，但增幅较小（表 4），其中仅有东部地区仪器设备的配置总数达到国家标准，中部、西部地区一直未达标。从仪器设备的分类项目来看，截至 2015 年，东部地区疾控机构只有健康教育器材的配置未达标，其余项目均达标；中部地区仅有车辆与冷链设备及器材的配置达到国家标准，其余 3 项均未达标（图 3）；而西部地区 5 年间所有项目的配置均滞缓，一直未达到国家标准。

表 4　2011 ~ 2015 年县区级不同地区疾控机构仪器设备配置状况

地区	2011 年		2012 年		2013 年		2014 年		2015 年	
	平均拥有件数	达标率（%）	平均拥有件数	达标率（%）	平均拥有件数	达标率（%）	平均拥有件数	达标率（%）	平均拥有件数	达标率（%）
国家标准	106	100.00	106	100.00	106	100.00	106	100.00	106	100.00
东部	114	107.55	141	133.02	131	123.58	131	123.58	138	130.19
中部	57	53.77	61	57.55	67	63.21	69	65.09	68	64.15
西部	43	40.57	45	42.45	47	44.34	48	45.28	51	48.11

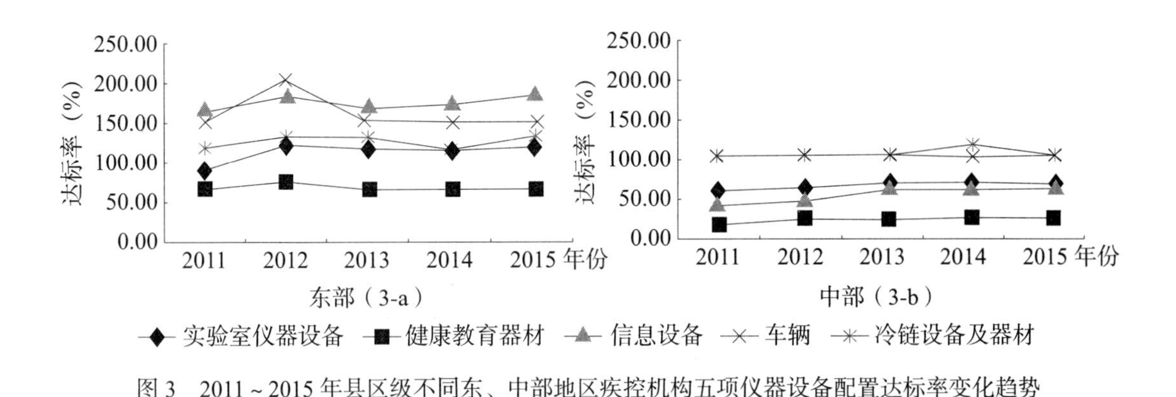

图 3　2011～2015 年县区级不同东、中部地区疾控机构五项仪器设备配置达标率变化趋势

3. 讨论

受 2003 年“非典”的影响，国家加大了对各级疾控机构建设的投入[6]。仪器设备的投入是疾控机构建设的基础，是提升疾控工作能力的关键一环[7]。2011～2015 年间全国各级、各地区的疾控机构仪器设备平均拥有数量与达标率总体呈逐年增加的趋势，可见经过国家不断对疾控机构建设发展的投入，我国疾控机构硬件设备建设已初见成效。但仍需要进一步有针对性的资金投入和配置规划。

3.1　不同级别疾控机构仪器设备配置达标情况存在差异

从“非典”起在十几年的疾控机构建设后，2011～2015 年省级、地市级、县区级疾控机构仪器设备配置的达标水平存在较大差异。我国省、地市、县区各级别间由于不同的行政区划，拥有不同的经济水平和资源条件，同样卫生资源分布也存在一定的差异[8]。对于具有公共卫生职能的疾控机构来说，不同层级的硬件设施资源配置也存在不均衡的现象。因此未来国家仍需加大对县区级疾控机构仪器设备的配置投入，同时要了解各级疾控工作实际需求，补充不足时也要避免资源过剩。除了国家的宏观调控，仍需各级政府制定相应的疾控建设规划，把握本地的疾控硬件配置情况，做出合理的调整[9-13]。

3.2　不同地区疾控机构仪器设备配置达标情况存在差异

省级东、中、西部三个地区疾控机构仪器设备的配置总量都超过国家标准；地市级东部和中部地区已达标，但西部地区还未达标；县区级仅东部地区达标，中部和西部地区都未达标。我国西部地区对基本公共卫生服务需求优先度高于东、中部地区，但卫生资源充沛度明显东部偏好于中、西部地区[14]。在疾控硬件设施资源这一点上，也证实了西部地区（地市、县区级）疾控机构存在不足。我国曾于 2003 年重点增加了专项资金用于支持中西部地区疾病控制机构建设[15]，经过多年的发展后，西部地区仍有所欠缺，因此还需加大对地市、县区两级西部地区疾控机构仪器设备的配置，尽力消除西部地区公共卫生工作中供需不平的现象。

3.3 不同类别仪器设备配置的达标情况存在差异

不同级别和地区疾控机构有不同种类的配置缺乏情况。除了地市和县区级西部地区整体设备配置缺乏外，综合来看，地市和县区级普遍对健康教育器材的配置匮乏情况较为严重。健康教育在促进疾控机构文化建设和慢性病防控工作中起着重要作用[16, 17]，因此健康教育器材配置的重要性不可忽视。今后国家和各级政府应按各级别、地区仪器设备相应缺乏情况，给予相关设备的资金投入。每一类仪器设备都有各自的职能任务，只有实现全部配置到位，才能增强疾控机构的综合能力。

综合研究结果与疾控机构的工作现状，我国仍应逐步加大对基层疾控体系的硬件设施建设，尤其是县区级、中西部地区的疾控机构。仪器设备作为疾控机构能力建设的基础，其合理配置理应受到广泛的重视。但是，加大财政投入力度来配置各疾控机构的仪器设备并不是盲目追求使其数量增加，而是要遵循疾控中心建设标准，坚持科学、合理、经济、适用的原则来完善疾控机构硬件设施体系。还要加强仪器设备管理和提高使用效率，使我国各级疾控机构都能够更好的发挥工作职能[18]。加强公共卫生人员队伍建设，提升工作人员技术、管理等整体素质，促进疾控工作规范化的同时也能进一步保证仪器设备合理使用[19]。

参考文献

[1] 蒋珊，庹晓莉，曾伟，等.2014 年成都市疾病预防控制机构能力建设情况分析 [J]. 现代预防医学，2016，43（6）：1044-1046.

[2] 隋红玉. 我国基层疾控机构的建设问题研究 [D]. 济南：山东大学，2015.

[3] 卢亮平，郑正红，罗成旺，等. 实验室仪器设备配置与科研、教育和疾病控制能力建设分析 [J]. 中国公共卫生，2013，29（10）：1515-1517.

[4] 罗智敏，王晓娟，陈瑾，等. 湖北省疾控机构实验室硬件建设现况 [J]. 公共卫生与预防医学，2014，25（6）：126-128.

[5] 邱延超. 提高石家庄市疾病预防控制机构管理效率对策研究 [D]. 保定：河北大学，2016.

[6] 于竞进，于明珠，苏海军，等. 中国疾病预防控制体系建设策略和落实效果 [J]. 中国公共卫生管理，2007，23（2）：98-101.

[7] 周晓红，胡薇薇，寿钧，等. 仪器设备配置与疾病预防控制中心能力建设分析 [J]. 浙江预防医学，2016（6）：646-648.

[8] 王德银，张馨予，王耀刚. 我国 31 个省、市、自治区卫生资源配置分析与评价 [J]. 中国卫生经济，2014（8）：37-39.

[9] 杨绯，刘阳波. 宁夏疾控机构实验室能力建设与现状调查 [J]. 中国公共卫生，2014，30（2）：225-226.

[10] 钱智勇，李镠. 天津市区县疾病预防控制机构实验室能力建设现状 [J]. 中国卫生检验杂志，2016（17）：2576-2578.

[11] 王海红. 东营市疾病预防控制机构实验室能力建设现状分析 [D]. 济南：山东大学，2015.

[12] 文献英，周云，先德强，等. 绵阳市疾病预防控制机构能力建设现状分析 [J]. 预防医学情报杂志，2014（6）：487-90.

[13] 秦俊，陈莉，郑朝晖，等. 湖北省 2009 ~ 2013 年疾控绩效考核机构建设和实验室检验能力评价 [J]. 公共卫生与预防医学，2015，26（5）：61-63.

[14] 峗怡. 我国公共卫生资源配置的公平性评价研究：基于公平基准方法的实证分析 [J]. 中国卫生经济，2014（1）：32-34.

[15] 国家支持中西部地区疾病控制机构建设 [J]. 领导决策信息，2003（15）：13-13.

[16] 张文娴，黄明豪. 浅谈健康教育在促进疾病控制机构文化建设中的作用 [J]. 健康教育与健康促进，2014（1）：73-75.

[17] 郭田. 健康教育在慢性病防治中的角色及作用 [J]. 实用医技杂志，2014，21（4）：437-38.

[18] 郭传广，舒高亭. 加强疾控中心仪器设备管理，不断提高使用效率 [J]. 医院管理，2010，48（19）：110-111.

[19] 陈家斌，张芬，肖菁. 加强公共卫生队伍建设，促进疾控工作规范化管理 [J]. 公共卫生与预防医学，2013，24（4）：125.

2010～2015年新疆疾控机构人员专业学历变化趋势分析△

刘　芳，翟　屹，石文惠，何柳，吴　静

中国疾病预防控制中心，北京 102206
通讯作者：吴静，E-mail：wujingcdc@163.com

摘　要　目的　通过分析2010～2015年新疆省、市、县区各级疾控机构人员的专业学历状况，了解不同时间、不同层级新疆疾控机构的人力素质特点及其变化趋势，为客观评估新疆疾控机构能力和制定新疆地区人力资源发展规划提供依据。**方法**　通过全国疾病预防控制基本信息系统收集相关数据，运用SAS 9.4软件，以学历作为核心指标，分年度、机构级别进行描述和趋势分析。**结果**　2010～2015年，新疆整体及各级疾控机构本科及以上学历人员比例逐年上升，2015年新疆本科及以上学历比例为30.21%，大专及以下学历比例有所下降，人员结构不断得到优化。**结论**　2010～2015年新疆各级疾控机构人员专业素质均有所提高，但与全国平均水平仍有差距。

关键词　新疆；疾控机构；学历；专业素质；趋势

Analysis on the Change Trend of Education Backgrounds among Staff in Disease Control Institutions in Xinjiang from 2010 to 2015

Liu Fang, Zhai Yi, Shi Wenhui, He Liu, Wu Jing
Chinese Center for Disease Control and Prevention, Beijing 102206, China

Abstract　Objective　To understand the characteristics and change trend of the quality of human resource of different times and at varied levels in Xinjiang disease control institutions and to provide evidence for

△　本文发表于：中国公共卫生管理，2018，34（2）：182-184＋188.

objective assessment on the ability of Xinjiang disease control institutions as well as the plan of human resource development in this area, by analyzing the education backgrounds of staff in disease control institutions at Provincial, municipal and county levels in Xinjiang from 2010 to 2015. **Methods** Data were collected through China Information System for Disease Control and Prevention. According to years and levels of institutions, the data were described and its trend was analyzed by SAS 9.4 software, with education background as the core indicator. **Results** From 2010 to 2015, the proportion of staff with bachelor degree or above raised year by year in Xinjiang as a whole and at all levels of disease control institutions. The number reached 30.21% in Xinjiang overall. Meanwhile, the proportion of staff with college degree or below declined. The staff structure has been constantly optimized. **Conclusions** Professional quality of staff at all levels of disease control institutions in Xinjiang was improved from 2010 to 2015, while there is still a gap compared with the national average.

Key words Xinjiang; disease control institutions; education background; professional quality; trend

各级疾病预防控制机构是承担政府疾病预防与控制、突发事件卫生应急、食品安全与卫生监督技术支撑、保护公众生命健康等公共卫生职能的公益性事业单位，是辖区疾病预防控制工作的业务管理、技术支持中心[1]，各级疾控机构人员专业素质是保证疾控机构履行职责的关键。新疆维吾尔自治区是我国面积最大的省级行政区，面积166万平方公里，占国土总面积六分之一。

2009年国务院在《关于深化医药卫生体制改革的意见》中规定，要“全面加强公共卫生服务体系，提高公共卫生服务和突发公共卫生事件应急处置能力，促进城乡居民逐步享有均等化的基本公共卫生服务”[2]。2016年国务院《关于印发“十三五”深化医药卫生体制改革规划的通知》中提出，“到2020年，普遍建立比较完善的公共卫生服务体系”，“健全基本公共卫生服务项目和重大公共卫生服务项目遴选机制”[3]，这都对各级疾控机构人员的专业素质提出了更高要求。

本研究以学历作为专业素质的衡量指标，对2010～2015年新疆不同层级的疾控机构人员学历进行趋势分析，并与全国疾控机构人员学历情况进行对比，分析探讨新疆疾控机构人员学历水平，为客观评估新疆疾控机构人员专业能力和制定发展规划提供依据。

1. 对象与方法

1.1 对象

2010～2015年新疆省级、地市级、县区级疾控中心在册正式职工，不包含新疆生产建设兵团各级数据。

1.2 资料来源与方法

通过全国疾病预防控制基本信息年度报告系统收集基础信息。该信息报告系统覆盖全国所有省级、地市级、县区级疾控中心，由通过统一培训的专人在线填报[4]，每年及时上报率均超过90%，信息经过严格审查与核对，数据真实可靠。

1.3 分析方法

对原始数据库进行再次逻辑核对后，分不同年份、不同层级，对新疆疾控机构人员的人力资源信息进行统计学描述和趋势分析。所有分析均采用SAS 9.4软件和Excel 2010进行。

2. 结果

2.1 基本情况

2010年新疆各级疾控机构工作人员共有5 097人，2015年新疆各级疾控机构工作人员总人数为4 979人，省级、地市级和县区级人数分别为450人、1 244人和3 285人。2010~2015年，新疆疾控机构人数总体趋势稳定，略有下降。详见表1。

表1 2010~2015年新疆/全国各级疾控机构人员数量

	省级	地市级	县区级	合计
2010	521/12 227	1 337/36 924	3 239/132 801	5 097/181 952
2011	521/11 633	1 311/37 191	3 288/133 021	5 120/181 845
2012	488/11 855	1 264/37 163	3 270/134 692	5 022/183 710
2013	447/11 792	1 264/37 308	3 285/135 338	4 996/184 438
2014	450/11 423	1 296/36 983	3 323/132 479	5 069/180 885
2015	450/11 890	1 244/36 758	3 285/132 383	4 979/181 031

2.2 不同年份新疆疾控机构人员学历变化情况

从总体角度，2010~2015年新疆疾控机构本科及以上学历比例逐年上升，学历构成变化趋势基本与全国疾控机构学历构成变化趋势相同。2015年新疆本科及以上学历比例为30.21%。新疆研究生比例从2010年的1.77%上升到2015年的2.79%，涨幅为57.62%，是四种学历中涨幅最大的。

大专及以下学历比例逐年下降，但仍是新疆疾控机构学历构成主体，2015 年大专及以下学历比例为 69.79%。大专人员比例六年来基本持平。2010-2015 年新疆疾控机构人员大专以下比例由 35.90% 下降到 2015 年的 29.91%，下降了近 6 个百分点。

表 2　2010 ~ 2015 年新疆 / 全国疾控机构人员学历构成（%）

	研究生	大学	大专	大专以下
2010	1.77/2.90	22.82/23.40	39.51/34.46	35.90/39.24
2011	1.86/3.42	23.87/25.98	39.53/34.83	34.74/35.77
2012	2.05/3.86	24.23/27.47	39.67/34.86	34.05/33.81
2013	2.28/4.33	25.20/29.16	40.21/34.94	32.31/31.57
2014	2.45/4.77	26.59/30.75	40.01/34.84	30.95/29.64
2015	2.79/5.19	27.42/32.45	39.88/34.66	29.91/27.70

2.3　不同级别疾控机构人员学历构成情况

2010 ~ 2015 年新疆省级、地市级、县区级疾控机构，本科及以上学历比例均呈上升趋势。其中省级疾控机构本科及以上比例由 52.01% 提高到 60.23%，增长了 8 个百分点；地市级和县区区级疾控机构本科及以上比例也分别增长了 7.53 个百分点和 5.38 个百分点。2010 ~ 2015 年新疆省级、地市级、县区级疾控机构大专以下学历人员逐年下降，与全国各级机构变化趋势一致。详见表 3 ~ 表5。

2.3.1 新疆省级疾控机构人员学历变化情况　2010 ~ 2015 年新疆省级疾控机构研究生比例由 8.06% 到 11.56%，增加了 3.5 个百分点，同期全国疾控机构研究生比例平均水平增加了 10.76 个百分点。2015 年新疆省级疾控机构大专以下比例降低了 5.49 个百分点。详见表 3。

2.3.2 新疆地市级疾控机构人员学历变化情况　2010 ~ 2015 年新疆地市级疾控机构研究生比例由 2.84% 增加到 4.34%，增加了 2.5 个百分点。2010 ~ 2015 年新疆地市疾控机构大专以下比例由 32.61% 下降到 26.28%，下降了 6.33 个百分点。详见表 4。

2.3.3 新疆县区级疾控机构人员学历变化情况　2010 ~ 2015 年新疆县区级疾控机构人员大专及以下比重逐年下降仍是学历构成的主体，2015 年大专及以下所占比例为 76.56%。2010 ~ 2015 年新疆县区级疾控机构大专以下比例由 39.33% 下降到 32.97%，下降了 6.36 个百分点。详见表 5。

表 3　2010～2015 年新疆 / 全国省级疾控机构人员学历构成（%）

	研究生	本科	大专	大专以下
2010	8.06/15.69	43.95/41.38	24.95/21.7	23.04/21.23
2011	8.06/19.05	43.95/43.18	24.95/19.83	23.04/17.94
2012	9.63/20.42	46.72/43.99	22.95/19.12	20.70/16.47
2013	10.29/22.78	48.10/44.45	22.82/18.26	18.79/14.51
2014	11.56/25.32	48.67/45.18	22.22/17.01	17.55/12.49
2015	11.56/26.45	48.67/44.60	22.22/16.39	17.55/12.56

表 4　2010～2015 年新疆 / 全国地市级疾控机构人员学历构成（%）

	研究生	本科	大专	大专以下
2010	2.84/5.45	26.85/36.03	37.70/30.93	32.61/27.59
2011	2.90/6.43	28.68/38.58	37.15/30.16	31.27/24.83
2012	3.01/7.52	29.83/40.35	36.71/29.29	30.45/22.84
2013	3.72/8.48	31.49/42.33	36.55/28.40	28.24/20.79
2014	3.70/9.14	32.25/43.96	37.04/27.68	27.01/19.22
2015	4.34/10.11	32.88/45.59	36.50/26.92	26.28/17.38

表 5　2010～2015 年新疆 / 全国县区级疾控机构人员学历构成（%）

	研究生	本科	大专	大专以下
2010	0.31/1.02	17.75/18.23	42.61/36.62	39.33/44.13
2011	0.46/1.21	18.77/20.96	42.79/37.44	37.98/40.39
2012	0.55/1.4	18.72/22.46	43.30/37.79	37.43/38.35
2013	0.64/1.58	19.67/24.19	43.99/38.20	35.70/36.03
2014	0.72/1.78	21.40/25.81	43.58/38.38	34.30/34.03
2015	1/1.91	22.44/27.71	43.59/38.44	32.97/31.94

3. 讨论

3.1　主要发现及结论

从整体看，2010～2015 年间，新疆各级疾控机构人员数量略有减少，但人员结构不断优化，本科及以上学历人员比例逐年上升。与同期全国疾控机构平均水平相比，仍有一定差距。2015 年，新疆各级疾控机构本科及以上人员比例低于同期全国疾控机构平均水平，与西部地区相比，也仅相当于西部地区 2013 年平均水平 [5]。

从不同层级疾控机构看，近几年来，新疆各级疾控机构人才结构不断得到优化，学历层次均有所改善，各级疾控机构大专以下学历比例均呈下降趋势，本科及以上学历比例逐年增加。与全国相比，新疆各级疾控机构本科及以上学历比例及增长速度均不同程度低于相应全国疾控机构平均水平。2009 年卫生部《关于加强卫生人才队伍建设的意见》中指出，到 2012 年省级、地市级、县区级疾控机构本科及以上学历人员比例分别为 65%、50%、35% 以上 [6]。2015 年新疆省级、地市级、县区级疾控机构本科及以上人员学历比例分别为 60.23%、37.22%、23.44%，距离文件要求还有一定差距。同时考虑到新疆地区慢性心肺疾病现况和发展趋势，为了更好地实现医防结合、有效控制，必须在疾控机构配备更多的相关专业人员。

卫生部 2008 年《各级疾病预防控制中心基本职责》中对地市、县区级疾控机构职责进行了明确规定，县区级疾控中心承担着大量公共卫生监测、现场调查、突发事件应对等技术工作 [7]。新疆地区地广人稀，基层疾控机构工作任务量大，需要相应数量、水平的疾控机构工作人员与之相适应。因此，需要着力调整和优化地市、县区疾控机构人员队伍结构，引进高层次人才提高基层人员素质 [8, 9]。

3.2 政策建议

“十二五”以来，医改各项工作扎实推进，基本公共卫生服务项目和重大公共卫生服务项目不断拓展，对疾控机构提出了更高的要求。新疆地处我国西部边陲，面积广阔、地广人稀，新疆各级疾控机构背负着更多的工作量和职责。但从本文分析可以看出，近年新疆各级疾控机构的人员数量不增反降，而且本科及以上高学历人才比例的增长速度和增长幅度有限，与国家要求仍有一定距离。为更好地推动“十三五”期间医药卫生体制改革步伐，造福新疆地区人民群众，提高当地群众健康水平，一方面结合新疆实际情况，综合考虑辖区内服务人口数、人口密度、服务半径、交通条件等因素，合理规划新疆疾控机构卫生资源机构和布局，核定、增加人员编制数量 [10-12]。另一方面，加强现有队伍能力建设，充分发挥对口支援单位作用，通过培训、进修等多种形式提高现有疾控工作人员业务素质。做到“重心下沉，关口前移”，尤其要重视地市、县区基层疾控机构人才队伍结构优化，提高基层疾控机构战斗力。

3.3 局限之处

本文仅以学历作为表征专业人员素质的分析指标，尚存在一定的局限性，主要发现和结论仅供参考，还需要更多相关研究的进一步验证。

参考文献

[1] 卫生部. 疾病预防控制机构管理的若干规定 (征求意见稿) 公开征求意见的通知 [EB/OL]. (2012-01-10). http: //www. moh. gov. cn/publicfiles/business/htmlfiles/ mohzcfgs/s3578/201201/53914. htm.

[2] 中共中央，国务院. 中共中央国务院关于深化医药卫生体制改革的意见 [R]. 北京：国务院 , 2009.

[3] 国务院. 国务院关于印发“十三五”深化医药卫生体制改革规划的通知 [R]. 北京：国务院，2016.

[4] 杨洋，王松旺，张英杰，傅罡. 全国疾病预防控制中心人力资源现状分析 [J]. 中国数字医学，2013(10).

[5] 刘芳，吴静，陈骏籍，等. 2010-2013 年全国疾控机构人员专业学历变化趋势分析 [J]. 中国公共卫生管理，2015, 31(3).

[6] 卫生部，国家发展改革委，财政部，等. 卫生部关于加强人才队伍建设的意见 [R]. 北京：卫生部，2009.

[7] 卫生部疾控局. 各级疾病预防控制中心基本职责 [R]. 北京：卫生部疾控局，2008.

[8] 卫生部. 关于疾病预防控制体系建设的若干规定 (卫生部令第 40 号)[R]. 北京：卫生部，2005.

[9] 潘东霞，顾华，林峰，陈永弟，孙建中. 浙江省疾病预防控制中心人力资源现状调查 [J]. 实用预防医学，2013, 20(3).

[10] 侯鹏. 2009 ~ 2011 年新疆疾病预防控制机构人力资源现状调查分析 [D]. 新疆：新疆医科大学，2013 : 1-21.

[11] 热沙来提 • 阿不都克力木，路阳，麦尔当 • 力木，等. 新疆维吾尔自治区卫生人力资源现状分析 [J]. 医学与社会，2015, 28(9).

[12] 姜婷 , 李斌 . 新疆两地区卫生机构及卫生人力资源配置现状研究 [J]. 中国社会医学杂志 , 2015, 32(1).

会议论文摘要

Association of Obesity Types with the 10-year Coronary Heart Disease Risk in Tibet and Xinjiang Regions of China △

ZHENG Congyi, WANG Zengwu, CHEN Zuo, ZHANG Linfeng, WANG Xin, DONG Ying, WANG Jiali, SHAO Lan, TIAN Ye

Fuwai Hospital, Chinese Academy of Medical Sciences; Department of Prevention and Community Health, National Center For Cardiovascular Diseases Beijing 102308

Abstract **Objective** To investigate the association between types of obesity and 10-year coronary heart disease risk in a Tibetan and Xinjiang populations of China. **Methods** Using stratified multi-stage random sampling, We examined 7 631 populations aged 35 or oeder with international standardized examination in 2015-2016. There were 5 802 participants were eligible for analysis. **Results** The prevalence of general obesity, General obesity, visceral obesity and compound obesity were 0.53%, 12.62%, 10.08% and 42.35%, respectively. Out of all compound obesity, 58.65% (1441/2457)included all types of the obesity in our study. The 10-year coronary heart disease risk of man was higher than woman [(3.05 ± 4.14)% for man and (1.42 ± 2.37)% for woman, respectively] ($P < 0.000\ 1$). Compound obesity (30.16%) had the greatest percent of the highest 10-year coronary heart disease risk than central obesity (28.01%), visceral obesity (18.46%) and general obesity (19.35%). After adjustment for confounding factors, multivariate analysis found disease risk than central obesity (28.01%), visceral obesity (18.46%) and general obesity (19.35%). After adjustment for confounding factors, multivariate analysis found that compound obesity was associated with the greatest risk to the 10-year coronary heart disease risk (OR, 95%CI: 2.889, 2.525-3.305), more people with anomalous body mass index, (BMI) and waist circumstance, (WC) had greater risk (OR, 95%CI: 3.168, 2.730-3.677). **Conclusions** Obesity is prevalent in Tibet and Xinjiang regions of China. Male and compound obesity (especially both BMI and WC are abnormal) populations have a greater risk to 10-year coronary heart disease.

△ International Academy of Cadiclogy, Annual Scientific Sessions 2017, 22nd World Congress on Heart Diseases, 2017.

Association between Metabolic Syndrome with Left Ventricular Diastolic Function among 1 516 Adults in Tibet, China △

ZHENG Congyi, WANG Zengwu, CHEN Zuo, ZHANG Linfeng, WANG Xin, DONG Ying, WANG Jiali, SHAO Lan, TIAN Ye

Fuwai Hospital, Chinese Academy of Medical Sciences; Department of Prevention and Community Health, National Center For Cardiovascular Diseases Beijing102308

Abstract **Objective** To explore the association between metabolic syndrome and left ventricular diastolic dysfunction among Tibetan population of China. **Methods** We did a cross-sectional survey in a representative sample of 1516 Tibetans aged 35-86 years in 2015-16. The metabolic syndrome was defined according to the revised NCEP ATP Ⅲ criteria (2004) appropriated for Asian population. **Results** Totally 1516 participants (mean age: 52.16 ± 10.83 years, 62.14% females) were grouped according to the number of criteria satisfied: (1) Absent (0 criteria, n = 186, 12.27%); (2) Pre-metabolic syndrome (1-2 criteria, n = 930, 61.35%); and (3) Metabolic syndrome (⩾ 3 criteria, n = 400), the crude and age-standardized prevalence of metabolic syndrome were 26.38% (400/1516) and 22.42%. LV ejection fractions, left atrial diameter and LV diameter were similar among the three groups. After adjustment for confounding factors, multivariate analysis found that elevated blood pressure(OR, 95%CI: 1.490, 1.132-1.962), fasting blood glucose (OR, 95%CI: 1.714, 1.185-2.479) and abdominal obesity (OR, 95%CI: 1.912, 1.463-2.498) were significantly associated with increased risk of left ventricular diastolic dysfunction. Moreover, participants with metabolic syndrome had greater risk (OR, 95%CI: 2.245, 1.393-3.618). **Conclusions** Metabolic syndrome (high blood pressure and elevated blood glucose as the major contributors) population has a greater risk to left ventricular diastolic dysfunction independent of LV mass among Tibetans. These functional abnormalities may partially explain the increased cardiovascular morbidity and mortality associated with metabolic syndrome.

△ 第四届世界高血压大会，2017.

我国新疆、西藏地区居民肥胖类型与 10 年冠心病发病风险关系的研究△

郑聪毅，王增武，陈 祚，张林峰，王 馨，董 莹，聂静雨，王佳丽，邵 澜，田 野

中国医学科学院阜外医院，国家心血管病中心社区防治部，北京 102308

通信作者：王增武，Email：wangzengwu@foxmail.com

摘 要 目的 利用公益性行业科研专项“西藏与新疆地区慢性心肺疾病现状调查研究”的相关数据，分析新疆、西藏两地 35 岁及以上居民肥胖类型，并探讨肥胖类型与 10 年冠心病发病风险的关系，为制定西部地区包括冠心病在内的心血管疾病防治策略提供科学依据。**方法** 采用多阶段分层随机抽样的方法，共抽取新疆、西藏两地≥ 35 岁研究对象 7 631 名，其中 5 804 人纳入本研究分析。按照不同的肥胖特征将调查对象分为五类：①普通肥胖：腰围和内脏脂肪指数正常，但 BMI ≥ 28 kg/m^2；②腹型肥胖：BMI 和内脏脂肪指数正常，但腰围 > 90 cm（男）/85 cm（女）；③内脏肥胖：BMI 和腰围正常，但 VFA ≥ 100 或 VFI ≥ 10；④混合型肥胖：同时符合以上两种或三种类型肥胖标准；⑤非肥胖：以上三种肥胖类型标准均不满足。估计 10 年冠心病发病风险的方法为 2004 年发表的中国多省队列研究（Chinese Multi-provincial Cohort Study，CMCS）中 Framingham 校正均值和系数后的预测模型，公式中变量包括：年龄、血压水平、总胆固醇、高密度脂蛋白、是 / 否吸烟和是 / 否糖尿病六项评估指标。自然人群中的 10 年冠心病风险大多集中在 < 5%，故本文采用四分位法将 10 年冠心病发病风险由低至高分为四等级进行单因素和多元 Logistic 回归分析。**结果** 本研究实际纳入分析对象 5 802 人，其中男性 2 554 人（44.02%），平均年龄（53.16 ± 12.63）岁，汉族占 36.32%（2 107/ 5 802）。研究对象的普通肥胖、腹型肥胖、内脏肥胖和混合型肥胖患病率分别为 0.53%、12.62%、10.08% 和 42.35%。其中混合肥胖中同时满足三种肥胖类型诊断标准的研究对象占 58.65%（1 441/2 457）。男、女 10 年冠心病发病风险分别为（3.05 ± 4.14）% 和（1.42 ± 2.37）%（男性高于女性，$P < 0.000\ 1$）。混合型肥胖研究对象高等级冠心病发病风险所占比例为 30.16%，显著高于普通肥胖（19.35%）、腹型肥胖（28.01%）和内脏肥胖（18.46%）。Logistic 多因素分析模型中调整了年龄、性别、民族、饮酒、居住地海拔、受教育程度、农村 / 城镇户口、冠心病家

△ 第十九届中国南方国际心血管病学术会议，2017.

族史共 8 个 10 年冠心病发病风险预测模型变量之外的混杂因素，分析结果如图 2，混合型肥胖人群的 10 年冠心病发病风险高于其他肥胖类型（OR，95%CI：2.889，2.525 ~ 3.305），其中 BMI 和腰围两项指标均异常的研究对象 10 年冠心病风险更大（OR，95%CI：3.168，2.730 ~ 3.677）。**结论**　肥胖问题在我国新疆、西藏地区较为严重，男性、混合型肥胖（特别是 BMI 和腰围均异常）人群或是 10 年冠心病发病的高危人群。

我国新疆和西藏地区居民体重指数及腰围与10年冠心病发病风险关系的研究△

郑聪毅，王增武，陈　祎，张林峰，王　馨，董　莹，聂静雨，王佳丽，邵　澜，田　野

中国医学科学院阜外医院，国家心血管病中心社区防治部，北京 10238

通信作者：王增武，Email：wangzengwu@foxmail.com

摘　要　目的　冠心病和脑卒中是全球首要死因，在发展中国家，冠心病患病率与国家发展指数呈正比，2002～2014年中国冠心病病死率呈上升趋势。肥胖是冠心病重要的危险因素之一，近23%的冠心病是肥胖引起。本研究利用公益性行业科研专项“西藏与新疆地区慢性心肺疾病现状调查研究”的相关数据，探讨体重指数和腰围这两种常见肥胖指标与10年冠心病发病风险的关系，为制定我国西部地区有效预防和控制心血管疾病策略提供科学依据。**方法**　采用多阶段分层随机抽样的方法，共抽取新疆和西藏地区≥35岁研究对象7 631例，其中资料完整的5 737例纳入分析。体重指数分为3个等级组：A组＜24 kg/m^2、B组≥24～＜28 kg/m^2、C组≥28 kg/m^2；腰围分为3个等级组：Ⅰ组＜85（男）/80（女）cm、Ⅱ组≥85～＜90（男）/≥80～＜85（女）cm、Ⅲ组≥90（男）/85（女）cm。估计10年冠心病发病风险的方法为2004年发表的中国多省队列研究（Chinese Multi-Provincial Cohort Study，CMCS）中Framingham校正均值和系数后的预测模型，公式中变量包括：年龄、血压水平、总胆固醇、高密度脂蛋白、是/否吸烟和是/否糖尿病6项评估指标。自然人群中的10年冠心病风险大多集中在＜5%，故本文采用四分位法将10年冠心病发病风险由低至高分为四等级进行单因素和多元Logistic回归分析。**结果**　体重指数C组和腰围Ⅲ组的研究对象高血压、高总胆固醇、低HDL-C和糖尿病比例较大（均$P<0.01$）。体重指数各等级组的10年冠心病发病风险绝对值随腰围水平的增加而增加（趋势检验$P<0.000\,1$）；对于腰围水平低的对象，其体重指数水平越高，冠心病发病风险绝对值越高（趋势检验$P=0.000\,6$）。多因素Logistic分析调整了性别、年龄、民族、饮酒、居住地海拔、受教育程度、农村/城镇户口、冠心病家族史8个10年冠心病发病风险预测模型变量之外的混杂因素，结果表明，对于同一体重指数（或腰围）等级的研究对象，其10年冠心病发病风险随腰围（或体重指数）水平的增加而增加（OR值的趋势检验

△　中国心脏大会（CHC）[1]，2017.

$P < 0.05$）；与体重指数 A 组且腰围Ⅰ组的研究对象比较，体重指数 C 组且腰围Ⅲ组的冠心病发病风险最大（OR，95%CI：4.191，3.578 ~ 4.909）。**结论**　新疆、西藏两地居民 BMI 和腰围是 10 年冠心病发病风险的独立影响因素，BMI 和腰围同时处于较高水平者或是 10 年冠心病发病的高危人群。

Comparison of Visceral and Body Fat Indices and Anthropometric Measures for Predicting the Clustering of Cardiometabolic Risk Factors by Gender among Adults in Tibet and Xinjiang Regions △

WANG Jiali, WANG Zengwu, CHEN Zuo, ZHANG Linfeng, WANG Xin, DONG Ying, ZHENG Congyi, SHAO Lan, TIAN Ye

Fuwai Hospital, Chinese Academy of Medical Sciences; Deparlment of Prevention and Community Health, National Center For Cardiovasular Diseases, Beijing 102308

Abstract **Objective** To compare the efficiency of bioelectrical indices (percentage body fat, PBF; visceral fat index, VFI) and various anthropometric measures (body mass index, BMI; waist circumference, WC; waist-to-height ratio, WHtR) in detecting the clustering of cardiometabolic risk factors (CCRF) among population aged 35-80 years in Tibet and Xinjiang area. **Method** We conducted the community-based cross-sectional survey during 2015 to 2017 in 13 sample sites selected by stratified multistage random sampling method from Tibet and Xinjiang area. Totally 7 564 residents aged 35-80 years were included and 5 558 (73.48%) participants were eligible for analysis. CCRF was defined by the existence of 2 or more of high blood pressure, hyperglycemia, high TG level, and high HDL-C level. **Results** The prevalence of clustering was 18.33%. In both genders, VFI and PBF tended to rise with age (all $P < 0.05$). However, for each age-specific group, women consistently had significantly greater PBF than men (all $P < 0.01$)and men had considerably higher VFI (all $P < 0.01$). Both PBF and VFI were significantly associated with CCRF. The area under the ROC curves (AUCs) for BMI, WC, WHtR, PBF, and VFI, respectively, were 0.673, 0.683, 0.665, 0.627, and 0.672 in men and 0.649, 0.664, 0.670, 0.643, and 0.669 in women. In men, AUCs for VFI in detecting CCRF was not significantly higher than that for BMI, WC, and WHtR; in women, AUCs for VFI was significantly higher than that for BMI ($P < 0.01$), but not for WC and WHtR; however, PBF had the lowest AUCs in both gender. Additionally, BMI yielded the greatest Youden

△ 13th Asian-Pacific Congress of Hypertension 2017.

index in identifying CCRF in men (0.27) and VFI yielded the greatest in women (0.26), respectively. Optimal cutoffs for VFI were 12 and 9 in men and women, respectively. **Conclusions** VFI is a better screening tool for identifying CCRF in women than BMI, but not superior to BMI in men.

Association between Low Pulmonary Function and Metabolic Syndrome in Xinjiang and Tibet Adults △

WANG Jiali, WANG Zengwu, CHEN Zuo, ZHANG Linfeng, WANG Xin, DONG Ying, ZHENG Congyi, SHAO Lan, TIAN Ye

Department of Prevention and Community Health, National Center for Cardiovascular Diseases, Fuwai Hospital, Chinese Academy of Medical Sciences; Beijing, 102308, China

Abstract **Objective** To evaluate the association between impaired lung function and metabolic risk factors among adults in Tibet and Xinjiang area. **Method** We conducted the community-based cross-sectional survey during 2015 to 2017 in 13 sample sites selected by stratified multistage random sampling method from Tibet and Xinjiang area. The study population included 3 824 subjects (age ≥ 35 years) who underwent spirometry test for lung function. We analyzed the association of lung function impairment with metabolic syndrome components using multiple linear regression and also analyzed the association of metabolic syndrome with restrictive and obstructive spirometry pattern using multiple logistic regression adjusted for sex, age, smoking, and the other covariates. **Results** Waist circumference, systolic blood pressure, and triglyceride were associated with forced vital capacity (FVC); and only triglyceride was so with forced expiratory volume in 1 second (FEV_1), but not with FVC and FEV_1/FVC ratio. The odds ratio of metabolic syndrome for restrictive spirometry pattern (FVC < 80%, FEV_1/FVC > 0.7) was 1.453(95% confidence interval, 1.020–2.070), and that for obstructive spirometry pattern (FEV1/FVC < 0.7) was 1.032 (95% confidence interval, 0.760 – 1.395) after adjustment for covariates. **Conclusions** Lung function impairment in the general population is associated with metabolic syndrome, especially the restrictive spirometry pattern.

△ 第四届世界高血压大会，2017.

我国新疆、西藏地区 35 岁及以上人群身体脂肪率、内脏脂肪指数与心脏代谢性危险因素聚集的关系[△]

王佳丽，陈　祚，张林峰，王　馨，董　莹，聂静雨，郑聪毅，邵　澜，田　野，王增武

中国医学科学院阜外医院，国家心血管病中心社区防治部　北京．102308

通讯作者：王增武，E-mail：wangzengwu@foxmail.com

摘　要　目的　肥胖与心血管疾病危险因素及其聚集密切相关，目前普遍采用体重指数和腰围作为评价肥胖及内脏脂肪蓄积的指标。近年有研究提示生物电阻抗测量指标包括身体脂肪率（body fat percentage，BFP）和内脏脂肪指数（visceral fat index，VFI）对代谢性危险因素及其聚集的预测效果可能更优。本研究利用西藏与新疆地区慢性心肺疾病现状调查研究中 35 岁及以上人群数据探讨 BFP、VFI 与心脏代谢性危险因素聚集的关系及预测价值。**方法**　2016 年期间，采用分层多阶段随机抽样，选取新疆西藏地区 35 岁及以上调查对象 7 571 人进行问卷调查、体格检查和实验室检测，有效数据 5 643 人（74.53%）。采用多因素 Logistic 回归分析 BFP、VFI 与代谢性危险因素聚集的关系，受试者工作特征（ROC）曲线分析并比较 2 项指标对危险因素聚集的预测价值。心脏代谢性危险因素聚集定义为高血压、糖尿病、高甘油三酯血症、低高密度脂蛋白胆固醇血症 4 项中同时存在 2 项或 2 项以上。**结果**　新疆西藏地区 35 岁及以上居民代谢性危险因素聚集患病率为 9.78%，男性和女性分别为 12.70% 和 7.36%（$P < 0.01$）。BFP、VFI 分别按照四分位数分组，不同 BFP、VFI 分组中高血压、糖尿病、高甘油三酯血症、低高密度脂蛋白胆固醇血症和危险因素聚集患病率差异显著（$P < 0.05$）。高血压和危险因素聚集患病率随着 BFP 水平的升高而增加（均 $P < 0.05$）；4 项危险因素及其聚集的患病率均随着 VFI 水平升高而增加（均 $P < 0.05$）。多因素 Logistic 回归分析显示，调整性别、年龄、民族、吸烟、饮酒、教育程度、职业劳动强度和海拔后，随着 BFP 或 VFI 水平升高，BFP 或 VFI 与危险因素聚集关联的 OR 值增大。以 BFP 为 5.0% ~ 27.0% 组 OR 值为 1，BFP 为 27.1% ~ 31.7%、31.8% ~ 36.6% 和 36.7% ~ 50.0% 时，危险因素聚集患病风险分别为 1.15 倍（OR = 1.15，95%CI：0.86，1.54）、1.48 倍（OR = 1.48，95%CI：1.05，2.07）和 1.72 倍（OR = 1.72，95%CI：1.10，2.68）；以 VFI 为 1 ~ 6 组的 OR 值为 1，VFI 为 7 ~ 9、10 ~ 13 和 14 ~ 30 时，危险因素聚集患病风险分别为 1.20 倍（OR = 1.20，95%CI：0.81，1.79）、1.91 倍（OR = 1.91，95%CI：1.30，

△　中国心脏大会（CHC），2017.

2.80）和3.91倍（OR = 3.91，95%CI：2.64，5.77）。受试者工作特征（ROC）曲线分析，BFP、VFI预测危险因素聚集的ROC曲线下面积分别为0.55（95%CI：0.53～0.56）、0.70（95%CI：0.68～0.71），差异有统计学意义（$P < 0.01$）。**结论** 新疆西藏地区35岁及以上人群中，BFP和VFI水平均与心脏代谢性危险因素聚集有关，VFI对危险因素聚集的预测价值较好。提示在对肥胖及相关心血管代谢性疾病综合防治中，身体脂肪含量及脂肪分布均不容忽视。

Spirometric Reference Values for Tibet Residents Aged 15–98 Years △

GUO Yanfei[1*], XING Zhenzhen[1], CHAI Di[1], LIU Weiming[1], WANG Yuxia[1], TONG Yaqi[1], CUI Jia[1], TAN Xiaoming[1], SUN Tieying[1], WANG Chen[2]

1. Department of Pulmonary and Critical Care Medicine, Beijing Hospital, National Centre for Gerontology, Beijing, China; 2. Center for Respiratory Diseases, China-Japan Friendship Hospital; National Clinical Research Center for Respiratory Diseases, Beijing, China

* Corresponding author

Abstract **Background** Normal spirometric values and prediction equations are largely unknown for Tibet residents. This study aimed to determine spirometric values and establish prediction equations for healthy Tibet residents. **Methods** This prospective cross-sectional study enrolled 2909 healthy, nonsmoking Tibetans aged 15–98 years. A multistage cluster sampling strategy was used for sample selection. Anthropometric and spirometric data from six different urban and rural areas were obtained. Age stratification and the male to female ratio were highly considered. Student's t-test was used to obtain normal reference values based on sex and altitude. Multiple linear regression was used to establish prediction equations. **Results** The study was conducted between February 2015 and August 2016 in Tibet. Normal reference values of anthropometric data, such as age, height, and weight based on sex and altitudes, showed significant differences ($P < 0.01$). Additionally, prediction equations with age, height, and weight were established for FVC and FEV_1 between different genders and altitudes, respectively. Height and weight had positive effects on the equations, while age had negative relationships. **Conclusions** This study for the first time provides reference values for demographic characteristics and spirometry data for healthy Tibetans, with spirometry reference prediction equations based on sex and altitude.

△ The Asian Pacific Society of Respirology (APSR) Congress, 2017.

高海拔地区成人肺功能分布研究△

郭岩斐[1*]，邢珍珍[1]，柴　迪[1]，刘伟明[1]，王玉霞[1]，仝亚琪[1]，崔　佳[1]，谭晓明[1]，孙铁英[1]，王　辰[2]

1. 北京医院 / 国家老年医学中心呼吸与危重症医学科，北京 100730；2. 中日友好医院 / 国家呼吸疾病临床医学研究中心呼吸与危重症医学科，北京 100029

摘　要　目的　调查高海拔地区 15 岁以上人群的肺功能情况，分析年龄、性别、体重、身高、海拔等因素对肺功能影响，确定高海拔地区成人肺功能参考值分布及正常预计值方程。**方法**　收集西藏地区 15 岁以上健康人群基本情况、呼吸问卷、X 线胸片及全套肺功能资料，根据合格肺功能结果筛选出健康非吸烟人群。基于不同性别及海拔界限为 3 800 m 时，研究分析年龄、身高、体重、第 1 秒用力呼气量和用力肺活量的分布，并以年龄、身高、体重作为参数进行多元逐步线性回归分析，获得成人肺功能正常预计值方程。**结果**　研究纳入 15 ~ 98 岁健康非吸烟受试者 2 909 例（男性 1 025 例，女性 1 884 例）。不同性别和海拔下的年龄、身高及体重分布状况存在显著性差异（$P < 0.01$）。肺功能指标 FEV_1 和 FVC 在不同性别间存在显著性差异，在海拔高度 > 3 800 m 时显著高于低海拔地区。肺功能预计值方程显示，肺功能指标 FEV_1 和 FVC 与身高、体重呈正相关，与年龄呈负相关，其中与身高相关性最强。**结论**　本研究提供了高海拔地区成人正常肺功能参考值，并根据年龄、身高及体重建立了高海拔地区肺功能预计值方程。

△　第十八次全国呼吸病学学术会议，2017.

高海拔地区慢性阻塞性肺疾病患病率及其相关危险因素分析△

郭岩斐[1*]，邢珍珍[1]，柴　迪[1]，刘伟明[1]，王玉霞[1]，仝亚琪[1]，崔　佳[1]，谭晓明[1]，孙铁英[1]，王　辰[2]

1. 北京医院 / 国家老年医学中心呼吸与危重症医学科，北京 100730；2. 中日友好医院 / 国家呼吸疾病临床医学研究中心呼吸与危重症医学科，北京 100029

摘　要　目的　明确高海拔地区慢性阻塞性肺疾病的患病率及其主要危险因素。**方法**　通过多阶段整群随机抽样对西藏 6 个城乡地区 15 岁以上居民进行调查，内容包括基本资料、呼吸问卷、体格检查、X 线胸片及全套肺功能。以支气管舒张试验后第 1 秒钟用力呼气容积（FEV_1）/ 用力肺活量（FVC）< 70% 作为慢性肺部疾病（COPD）的诊断标准。**结果**　调查资料完整且肺功能检查合格的 3 871 例人群中，总体 COPD 患病率为 11.06%，其中 40 岁以上人群患病率为 14.86%，40 岁以下为 7.64%，在不同年龄上患病率存在显著性差异（$P < 0.05$）。高于 3 800 m 海拔地区人群患病率为 9.26%，低于 3 800 m 海拔地区人群患病率为 12.26%，不同海拔高度上患病率差异性存在统计学意义（$P < 0.05$）。多元回归分析显示年龄、低体重指数、室内吸入性因素及海拔高度可能与慢阻肺患病风险相关。**结论**　高海拔地区慢阻肺患病率高，经济负担重，迫切需要加强防治。

△　第十八次全国呼吸病学学术会议，2017.